No Real Choice

Families in Focus

Series Editors,
Naomi R. Gerstel, University of Massachusetts, Amherst
Karen V. Hansen, Brandeis University
Nazli Kibria, Boston University
Margaret K. Nelson, Middlebury College

For a list of all the titles in the series, please see the last page of the book.

No Real Choice

~

How Culture and Politics Matter
for Reproductive Autonomy

KATRINA KIMPORT

Rutgers University Press

New Brunswick, Camden, and Newark, New Jersey, and London

Library of Congress Cataloging-in-Publication Data
Names: Kimport, Katrina, 1978– author.
Title: No real choice: how culture and politics matter
for reproductive autonomy / Katrina Kimport.
Description: New Brunswick: Rutgers University Press, [2022] | Series: Families
in focus | Includes bibliographical references and index.
Identifiers: LCCN 2020057863 | ISBN 9781978817913 (paperback) |
ISBN 9781978817920 (cloth) | ISBN 9781978817937 (epub) |
ISBN 9781978817944 (mobi) | ISBN 9781978817951 (pdf)
Subjects: LCSH: Abortion—United States. | Abortion—Political aspects—
United States. | Abortion—Social aspects—United States. |
Abortion—Government policy—United States.
Classification: LCC HQ767.5.U5 K56 2022 | DDC 362.1988/800973—dc23
LC record available at https://lccn.loc.gov/2020057863

A British Cataloging-in-Publication record for this book is available from the
British Library.

♾ The paper used in this publication meets the requirements of the American
National Standard for Information Sciences—Permanence of Paper for Printed
Library Materials, ANSI Z39.48-1992.

www.rutgersuniversitypress.org

Manufactured in the United States of America

Contents

No Real Choice

1

No Real Choice

Sylvia, a twenty-four-year-old Black woman in Maryland, never wanted to have children.[1] She grew up with lots of young cousins and decided early on that she did not want to be a parent. This certainty softened over time and, when she was twenty-one, Sylvia had a daughter. It was not something she expected, but she was happy about it and devoted to her daughter. Indeed, while I interviewed her by phone, she invited her now-three-year-old daughter to say hello to me and introduce the doll she was playing with. When she was pregnant with her daughter, Sylvia sought to schedule a tubal ligation—a sterilization—after the birth. She only wanted one child. Her doctor, however, refused, insisting that she would change her mind about wanting more children. A little over two years later, in a new relationship, Sylvia became pregnant again. Even as she delighted in her daughter and was committed to her boyfriend, her desire not to have more children remained. Sylvia and her boyfriend had been using contraception. Both were shocked when Sylvia discovered this pregnancy, and neither felt ready to care for a new baby. They thought about abortion.

In the contemporary social narrative of pregnancy decision making, Sylvia was deciding among her "options": end the pregnancy or continue it, either then parenting or placing the baby for adoption. This rendering of the key question Sylvia was facing is

---

1. Sylvia and all the other respondent names in this book are pseudonyms.

remarkably widespread. Despite rampant political and social contention over abortion in the United States, people with opposing views generally agree that pregnant people choose between abortion and continuing the pregnancy. This construction of the choice pregnant people face rests on a few assumptions. For one thing, it constructs the decision as *between* two specific pregnancy outcomes: the pregnant person chooses either to end or to continue the pregnancy. For another, it constructs these outcomes as interrelated and mutually exclusive: choosing abortion means *not* choosing to continue the pregnancy, and vice versa. In many ways this makes logical sense—one cannot both abort and continue the same pregnancy—but these two assumptions collectively blur the distinction between pregnancy *outcomes* and the decision-making *question* that leads to an outcome. Just because the outcomes for a pregnancy are mutually exclusive and binary does not mean that the question pregnant people face is one of choosing between two binary outcomes. What if that was not the question Sylvia was facing?

In describing her thinking about what she wanted to do about her pregnancy, Sylvia kept coming back to her feelings about abortion. Her pregnancy decision making, in practice, was engaged with the question, Could she choose abortion? She was not, in other words, simply choosing between abortion and continuation. Sylvia explained that she felt that choosing abortion was irresponsible, that having an abortion was refusing to accept the "consequences" of having sex. She believed that abortion was not moral. She also recounted how physically difficult she had found an earlier miscarriage. Recalling that difficulty, Sylvia anticipated that the experience of an abortion would be equivalently painful—or worse. She did not want to experience that pain. Layered onto these components of her decision making was a concern about the cost of an abortion. Less than two months into her pregnancy, Sylvia lost her job and her health insurance. Without insurance, Sylvia expected to have to pay out of pocket for an abortion. And without a job, she had other immediate and acute financial concerns, including paying her rent and feeding her child. In effect, Sylvia was not deciding between having an abortion and continuing her pregnancy. She was deciding whether she could have an abortion, given a series of constraints.

By the end of her first trimester, Sylvia knew that she could not choose abortion. She reasoned that she could not afford an abortion. She also recognized that she could not imagine choosing a pregnancy outcome she thought of as immoral and as signaling irresponsibility. Moreover, she was fearful of what the physical experience of an abortion would be. Unable to choose abortion, she said of continuing the pregnancy and having another child, "I know it's going to be hard." She worried about managing her diagnosed clinical depression and anxiety, both in general and specifically during pregnancy, as her obstetrician had taken her off her current antidepressant because of its negative effects on fetal development. She worried that her three-year-old would feel jealous of a new baby. She worried that her romantic relationship would not survive a newborn, especially as her boyfriend was unenthusiastic about becoming a parent. Without a job, she worried she would not be able to financially provide for her daughter and herself, let alone for a new baby. And these worries persisted even as she determined she could not choose abortion. While she knew she would not have an abortion for this pregnancy, she pointedly had not chosen to have a baby. Her pregnancy outcome was the upshot of her answering the question of whether she could choose abortion—not a question of choosing between abortion and having a baby.

Yet, from the outside, the constraints on Sylvia's ability to make a pregnancy choice were not obvious. From the outside, in continuing her pregnancy, Sylvia behaved just like someone who decided she wanted a baby. But Sylvia still did not want another child. This is a subtle and perhaps confusing phenomenon: Sylvia did not want to have a baby, but neither was she able to choose abortion. The result of those two seemingly contradictory desires was that she was resigned to continuing her pregnancy.

I interviewed Sylvia as part of a project that sought to understand why pregnant people consider but do not obtain an abortion. In Sylvia's case, building out from the specifics of her circumstances, she considered but did not obtain an abortion because she felt unable to choose abortion—and why she felt unable to do so rested on structural obstacles (like the cost of abortion), cultural narratives (including that abortion is immoral and irresponsible), and her own healthcare experience of miscarriage. Sylvia did not choose abortion because of social constraints, not because she wanted to have a baby. If at least some pregnant people are experiencing something similar, we are misunderstanding their reproductive decision making. And we are misunderstanding it because we are failing to recognize how, and for whom, pregnancy decision making is constrained.

In this book, drawing on the candid and affecting accounts of women like Sylvia who considered but did not obtain an abortion, I demonstrate that Sylvia was not alone in being unable to choose abortion. I show that pregnant people are making decisions about their pregnancies in a context shaped by—and, more pointedly for the women described in this book, constrained by—structural and cultural factors and their own embodied experience. The question they grapple with is, Given the structural and cultural obstacles to abortion they face, can they choose abortion? For the women I interviewed for this book, the answer was no. Abortion, for them, was unchooseable. They had no real choice.

In the following chapters, I show how the pregnancy outcomes of women like Sylvia are the product of structural barriers to abortion, antiabortion cultural narratives that make abortion socially difficult to choose, and previous negative experiences of health care. To make sense of their experiences of having no real choice, I offer the abortion as unchooseable framework. This framework posits that, for some pregnant people, abortion is not a real, available pregnancy outcome; it is unchooseable. When abortion cannot be chosen, the idea of reproductive "choice" is mythical: pregnant people continue their pregnancies, regardless of whether they want to have a baby. This matters not only in regard to the ability of women like Sylvia to choose abortion, but also for whether they are able to choose the circumstances under which they wish to parent, including their romantic relationship, their financial stability, and/or their community. Not being able to choose abortion curtails people's reproductive agency to make decisions about both pregnancy and parenting. By applying an abortion as unchooseable framework, this book exposes the constraints on some pregnant people's reproductive autonomy, identifying the patterns of race and class inequality underlying many of these constraints, and challenges their naturalization. It provides a counterframe to the normative assumption that all pregnant people who stay pregnant do so because they want to have a baby.

Considering but Not Obtaining an Abortion

Sylvia is not the only pregnant person to consider and not obtain an abortion. My colleagues and I, using the larger quantitative sample from which the interviews analyzed here were drawn, found that about 30 percent of women presenting for their first prenatal care visit at clinical sites in southern Louisiana and Baltimore, Maryland, had considered but not obtained an abortion for their current pregnancy (S. Roberts, Upadhyay, et al. 2018, 651). This book is about understanding why. Between June 2015 and June 2017, I interviewed fifty-eight of these pregnant women. Twenty-eight respondents were recruited in Louisiana, thirty in Maryland. Broadly, the interview respondents recruited from each state shared similar characteristics.

In addition to the interviewees from both states being demographically similar, the women I interviewed were demographically similar to women who *do* obtain abortions. This was not by design: the study set out to recruit pregnant people who had considered and not obtained an abortion, and we discovered that the people in our recruitment sites for whom this was true were low income or poor, and most were Black. Most were also already parenting at least one child. With over 850,000 abortions performed in the United States annually (Jones, Witwer, and Jerman 2019), there is no such thing as a typical abortion patient. It is notable, however, that abortion patients are disproportionately poor or low income and people of color, and that the majority of abortion patients have previously given birth (Jerman, Jones, and Onda

2016). Further illustrating the similarities between the interviewees and women who have abortions, nearly half (47%) of the respondents had obtained an abortion in the past; many of the interviewees *are* women who have abortions. But these women did not obtain an abortion for this pregnancy after considering one, suggesting that characteristics alone are insufficient to explain why they continued their pregnancies. (See the Methodological Appendix for more detail on study design, recruitment, and participant characteristics.)

Another explanation for why the women I interviewed continued their pregnancies after considering abortion could be that they differed from people who have abortions in their reasons for wanting to end this pregnancy. If the pregnant people who consider but do not obtain abortions are not demographically different from those who obtain abortions, patterned differences in their reasons for abortion could explain this divergent outcome: perhaps those who do not obtain an abortion are considering abortion for qualitatively different reasons.

Research conducted at different points over the past two decades finds consistency in the reasons abortion patients report for seeking abortion. Early work utilizing surveys of abortion patients identified concerns about how having a baby would change the woman's life, inability to afford a new baby, and their relationship, including not wanting to co-parent with the man involved in the pregnancy (Finer, Frohwirth, et al. 2005; Torres and Forrest 1988). These reasons were not mutually exclusive, and most participants cited more than one reason for wanting an abortion. More recently, social psychologist Antonia Biggs and colleagues, surveying nearly 1,000 women from across the United States, found that financial concerns were the most commonly cited reason for seeking an abortion (40%), followed by the timing of the pregnancy (36%), partner-related reasons (31%), and the needs of existing children (29%) (Biggs, Gould, and Foster 2013).

The reasons Sylvia, from the opening of the chapter, considered abortion fell into these categories. Indeed, the reasons all the women I interviewed considered abortion were in line with the reasons women who do obtain abortions report for seeking an abortion. As with the plurality of abortion patients in the study by Biggs, Gould, and Foster (2013), financial concerns weighed heavily on many respondents. For example, Valencia, a thirty-five-year-old Black and Mexican woman in Maryland, was the primary caregiver for her four children and her grandparents. She worried about bringing another child into her household with only her husband working for pay. Tara, a twenty-one-year-old Black woman in Maryland, similarly cited worries about financial instability, and recognized the dual difficulty and importance of providing such stability for a child, saying, "You have to sacrifice a lot of things, so your child can be good or okay and stuff like that." Tara worried about her ability to be the parent she wanted to be in her current financial situation.

Others explained that they considered abortion because of their existing children and career aspirations: Martina, a twenty-five-year-old Black woman in Maryland, had a four-month-old baby when she became pregnant and knew that having two small children would make it difficult to succeed on her desired career path. Citing the gendered pressures of parenthood, Martina explained, "I'm not saying that having a baby stops your career but when you have a baby, as a woman, your attention is focused on your kids." For women like Martina, having a(nother) baby would change their lives substantially, just as abortion patients in early surveys on their reasons for choosing abortion anticipated it would for them (Finer, Frohwirth, et al. 2005; Torres and Forrest 1988).

Several respondents worried that the timing of this pregnancy would interfere with their education goals. Alexis, an eighteen-year-old Black woman in Maryland, thought about abortion because she was just about to finish high school and worried about "not finishing school or something, or being a young mother. Not being the best mother I could be." Teresa, a twenty-six-year-old Black woman in Louisiana, too, was concerned that a pregnancy would prevent her from finishing her studies at a four-year college. She summed up, "I thought it came at the wrong time." These women wanted children, or more children, but not right now, as did a substantial portion of the participants in the 2013 study of abortion patients by Biggs, Gould, and Foster.

Additionally, as did nearly one-third of the Biggs, Gould, and Foster (2013) participants, many respondents reported that they considered abortion because of concerns about their partner or relationship issues. April, a twenty-year-old Black woman in Louisiana, thought about seeking an abortion because she felt embarrassed that she was pregnant and not married. She was also uncertain whether she wanted a continued relationship with her boyfriend, which she anticipated would happen if she had a child with him. Similarly, Trinity, a twenty-three-year-old Black woman in Maryland, considered abortion because of her relationship to the man involved in the pregnancy. He was the father of her six-year-old daughter but played no role in the child's life, which Trinity saw as hurting her daughter. Trinity knew that he would not act as a parent to a future child and explained, "I really don't want to bring another child into a situation where they will not have a dad." Sequitta, a thirty-eight-year-old Black woman in Maryland, had five children with two different fathers, and she found it challenging to coordinate parenting with two different men. Continuing this pregnancy would mean co-parenting with a third man. Sequitta was not opposed to this idea in principle, but she wanted any future co-parent to also be a long-term partner. She explained, "I do want another child, but I want another child by somebody I'm with and we can raise it together in the same household as a family. Not separate." This man was not interested in committing to her and her existing children.

Other respondents invoked more complicated life circumstances in explaining why they considered abortion. Sonja, a twenty-six-year-old Black woman in Louisiana, for instance, was homeless, living at her cousin's house with one of her daughters. She was unable to care for her older daughter, who was therefore currently living with a different family member. Recently, another relative had been murdered, and Sonja was still working through this trauma. When I asked her how abortion came to her mind, she said pointedly, "Because like I said, I'm not really stable. . . . I just felt like I couldn't bring no child into the world." On top of all this, the pregnancy came from a casual relationship with a man who was in a long-term relationship with somebody else. Before discovering she was pregnant, she had hoped to end her interaction with this man, but if she continued the pregnancy, that no longer felt possible: "If I have the baby, I'm going to have to deal with him because I have a child for him, and I'm not going to kick him out of his child's life."

Nicole's experience was complicated as well. Nicole, a twenty-five-year-old Black woman in Maryland, had broken up with her boyfriend right before she discovered her pregnancy. Their relationship had been going very badly. Both struggled with depression and had difficulty supporting each other emotionally. A few months after they moved in together the prior summer, Nicole's boyfriend was physically violent toward her. It was not the first time. As Nicole explained, "We have a lot of fights, a lot of arguments. It's just unhealthy. We both battle with depression and stress. . . . I don't think we can handle helping each other while trying to help ourselves." Ten months after moving in with her boyfriend, Nicole moved out to live with her parents—and then discovered she was pregnant. She considered seeking an abortion because she was not working, did not have her own place to live, and was ashamed to be pregnant when she was not married. Having a baby, for her, meant getting back together with a man she believed would continue to be violent toward her.

Other respondents considered abortion because they did not want any future children. Michelle, a thirty-six-year-old white woman in Louisiana, for example, had never wanted children. Shaquira, a twenty-six-year-old Black woman in Louisiana, only ever wanted one child—and she had him already. Samantha, a thirty-eight-year-old white woman in Maryland, was looking forward to her children enrolling in school so that she could re-enter the workforce after having stayed home with them for several years.

Khadijah, a twenty-nine-year-old Black woman in Maryland, had three children, aged nine, ten, and eleven, and was not anticipating "starting over," as she called it, with a new baby. Several respondents, like Noreen, a thirty-eight-year-old Black woman in Louisiana, commented, "I'm too old for this."

Still other respondents considered abortion because of their pregnancy-related health challenges. One had a history of severe postpartum depression, another of multimonth postpartum hospitalization for diabetic ketosis, and another of preeclampsia (three times) and a placental abruption. For health reasons, they did not want to experience a full-term pregnancy again.

While not all respondents' reasons for abortion fit neatly into the categories scholars have identified—and some spanned more than one category—they were all consistent with the reasons abortion patients report for seeking an abortion. This means that reasons for abortion cannot explain why some people consider but do not obtain abortions and others do obtain abortions. It could be that people varied in the strength of their reasons for abortion. Perhaps someone more ambivalent about continuing a relationship would be more likely to continue the pregnancy compared to someone who was very clear she did not want to raise a baby with her current partner. Research has not measured strength of reasons for abortion. A cursory review of the examples I share above, however, demonstrates that the women I interviewed were not equivocal in their reasons for considering an abortion. Michelle, for example, did not want any children and had four prior abortions. Her desire to remain childfree had not changed with this pregnancy. Nicole was certain her boyfriend would be violent toward her again if they had a child together, and she did not want to be abused. Valencia was already struggling to meet the needs of her household and knew that adding another child would stretch them beyond what they could do. Their experiences illustrate the difficulties of positing lack of desire or ambivalence as an explanation for why they did not obtain an abortion when other women offering similar reasons do obtain abortions.

The Problem with Reasons for Abortion

In terms of efforts to understand pregnant people's decision making, the lack of difference in reported reasons for abortion between the respondents and people who do obtain abortions belies an emphasis on reported reasons alone for understanding abortion decision making. A reasons framework, as sociologist Carrie Purcell (2015) notes, is rooted in framings of abortion as a public health or healthcare provision issue. As such, it can be useful in efforts to improve access to abortion and for evaluating experiences of care. Abortion care workers, for example, may be able to better tailor their care to patients by understanding at a personal level why people present for abortion care. But the utility of this information has limits and may have unintended consequences outside of care provision.

One way this occurs owes to the structure of a reasons framework: it privileges individualism in understanding social phenomena, undervaluing constraints and opportunities outside of the individual that may be consequential to their ability to present for abortion care. Attention primarily or exclusively to a person's reasons for abortion as explanatory of a pregnancy outcome fails to account for other factors recognized as central to health decision making. Indeed, robust health decision-making models include not only the individual's values, beliefs, and decisional conflict but also the perceptions of important others and the availability of the necessary resources to make and implement a health decision (O'Connor et al. 1998). A reasons framework inaccurately flattens the complexity of pregnancy decision making.

Given the limitations, both observable and conceptual, of a reasons framework and a demographic interpretation for understanding pregnancy decision making, I propose thinking through why the women I interviewed considered but did not obtain abortions by attending to the context in which their decision making took place. I start with the recognition that the women I spoke with lived in a social, economic, and emotional context with constraints.

And those constraints, I show, could render abortion unchooseable, meaning that these women considered and did not obtain an abortion because abortion was not a true option. In the next sections, I walk through three specific ways this could happen: structural barriers, the limits of cultural narratives, and negative prior experiences of health care.

Structures

Abortion in the United States is legal, following the 1973 U.S. Supreme Court decision in *Roe v. Wade*. That and subsequent decisions, however, allowed individual states to regulate abortion provision (Hull and Hoffer 2010). In practice, regulation has meant restriction, with antiabortion politicians seeking to regulate abortion out of a desire to prevent abortions (Hull and Hoffer 2010). While states passed a steady stream of regulations in the decades following *Roe*, the rate of state-level abortion restrictions introduced, passed, and signed into law increased dramatically in 2010 when Republicans achieved one-party control of both the legislative and executive branches in many states, and this high rate has persisted in the years since (Nash and Gold 2015; Nash 2020).

As a result, in parts of the United States, pregnant people face myriad obstacles to obtaining an abortion, from policies regulating access to care to difficulty finding a provider due to the organization of abortion provision. The regulation of abortion means that some women continue their pregnancies not because they want to have a baby but because they are unable to access abortion services. These structural obstacles can prevent pregnant people from obtaining the resources they need to implement a decision, one of three components of health decision making (O'Connor et al. 1998). Their decision for abortion, as well as their reason(s) for abortion, becomes moot, and does so without a concurrent decision to have a baby. People may continue their pregnancies, in other words, because abortion is unavailable rather than out of a desire to have a baby.

The women I interviewed in Louisiana faced a raft of policies regulating and restricting abortion access, while those in Maryland did not. During data collection from 2015 to 2017, Louisiana had numerous laws on the books restricting abortion (Guttmacher Institute 2018a). Among them, focusing on those targeting the pregnant person, Louisiana prohibited the use of public funds to pay for abortion care (with a handful of exceptions), banned abortion after twenty weeks postfertilization (with a handful of exceptions), required abortion patients to make two separate visits to the provider at least twenty-four hours apart, and mandated that all abortion patients receive a pre-abortion ultrasound scan, which the provider had to show and describe to the patient. The state had still more restrictions that were blocked from taking effect by the courts, including a law passed in 2014 requiring all abortion-providing physicians to have admitting privileges at a nearby hospital. In 2020, the U.S. Supreme Court ruled the admitting privileges law unconstitutional in *June Medical Services LLC v. Russo*.

Scholars have investigated the effects of similar laws in other states. An extensive body of research has examined the prohibition on the use of public funds to pay for abortion. This prohibition means that, in practice, Medicaid does not cover abortion, and thus it centrally affects the low-income and poor people who rely on Medicaid for health insurance. Pregnant people on Medicaid in Louisiana must pay out of pocket for abortion care. Although the cost of a first-trimester abortion has remained stable and, for outpatient health care, relatively low over the years, averaging just above $500 in 2014 (Jones, Ingerick, and Jerman 2018), the out-of-pocket costs of abortion can represent a substantial amount for many people. Public health scientist Sarah Roberts and colleagues show that, for low-income women, abortion costs can represent more than one-third of their monthly personal income (S. Roberts, Gould, et al. 2014). Abortions after the first trimester of pregnancy can cost substantially more, as the type of procedure used changes as gestation increases. Second-trimester and later abortions may also incur higher costs for travel because there are fewer providers of this care, and patients tend to have to travel longer distances to reach them (Fuentes and Jerman 2019; Jones, Ingerick, and Jerman 2018).

On the books, public insurance coverage bans like the one in Louisiana often have exceptions, allowing coverage for abortion when the pregnancy is the result of rape or incest or if the pregnant person's life is in danger. In practice, few pregnancies for which women seek an abortion fit these criteria. Research has found that only approximately 1 percent of pregnancies for which women seek an abortion are the result of rape (Biggs, Gould, and Foster 2013). Further, even when a pregnancy fits the exception criteria, implementing an exception can be very difficult as a consequence of the structure of abortion care provision, including because abortion-providing clinics may lack the infrastructure to accept Medicaid reimbursement (Kimport and Rowland 2017). Poor people in states that ban public funding of abortion have no real recourse.

Research shows that the absence of Medicaid coverage lowers the abortion rate. The now-classic analysis from public policy scholar Philip Cook and colleagues (1999) examined whether the absence of Medicaid funding affected the abortion rate in North Carolina. Between 1980 and 1994, North Carolina Medicaid paid for recipients' abortion care using a block grant. When the annual grant ran out of money, the state stopped funding abortion care. Drawing on this natural experiment, Cook and colleagues analyzed whether the existence—and subsequent nonexistence—of funding affected the state's abortion rate. They found that the lack of Medicaid funding did affect the abortion rate, demonstrating that some Medicaid recipients continued pregnancies they would have otherwise terminated because of the absence of state funds for abortion. Specifically, they estimated that had public funding been available, approximately one-third of pregnancies that were carried to term would have, instead, ended in abortion. Recent analyses of the impact of public funding bans using data from the quantitative portion of this study in Louisiana corroborate these findings (S. Roberts, Johns, et al. 2019). It bears stating that the power of this ban rests on another structure: poverty. The public insurance ban on abortion coverage is consequential because the people who depend on public insurance are struggling financially and cannot simply overcome the funding ban with their own money.

Louisiana is also at the forefront of a recent trend to reduce the legal gestational age for abortion, broadly banning abortion after twenty weeks postfertilization. These laws are squarely unconstitutional, conflicting with the precedent established in *Planned Parenthood v. Casey* that states cannot prohibit abortion before viability, generally accepted to occur twenty-two weeks postfertilization (Hull and Hoffer 2010). Constitutional or not, this law prevents pregnant people from legally obtaining an abortion in Louisiana after twenty weeks postfertilization. Public health scientist Ushma Upadhyay and colleagues have shown that gestational age limits on abortion provision result in more than 4,000 women in the United States being unable to obtain a wanted abortion every year—and this effect is pronounced for low-income and poor women, connecting this structural barrier to other disadvantaging structures (Upadhyay, Weitz, et al. 2014).

Other regulations on abortion in Louisiana, such as its two-visit requirement, mandatory pre-abortion ultrasound viewing, and state-mandated information provision, have also been studied in other settings. These laws are passed under the logic that people considering abortion need additional information and time to consider their abortion decision. Yet research on the impact of these laws suggests they have little effect on abortion outcomes at the point of receiving abortion care. Among pregnant people who presented for care under a seventy-two-hour waiting period in Utah, for example, few reported any decision conflict, and the vast majority proceeded to abortion (S. Roberts, Turok, et al. 2016). Likewise, under a mandatory pre-abortion ultrasound viewing law in Wisconsin, nearly all patients proceeded to abortion (Upadhyay, Kimport, et al. 2017). Intriguingly, my colleagues and I (Kimport, Johns, and Upadhyay 2018) show that mandatory viewing laws like the one in Wisconsin have differential effects on abortion patients by race. Specifically, whether Black women viewed or declined to view their ultrasound image was more greatly affected by the law than was white women's viewing behavior, posing the possibility that policy restrictions coerce some patients' decisional autonomy more than others'. Sociologist Alexa Solazzo (2019) also finds that waiting period and counseling laws are associated with an increase in the gestation at the time of abortion for Black women, but not for white women, illustrating another differential impact of restrictive laws by race. An increase in gestation can matter not only because it might push a pregnant person beyond the state's or facility's gestational age limit for abortion, but also because the cost of abortion increases with gestation, and what kind of abortion procedure is available changes with gestation. Medication abortion, for example, is only available early in pregnancy; delays in access to care may mean that a pregnant person who desires a medication abortion cannot have one.

From these studies, in other words, we know that at least some of the restrictions in Louisiana matter for whether pregnant people obtain the abortion they want. And research suggests that the presence of multiple restrictions may reinforce and augment their individual negative impact on the ability to obtain an abortion (Jerman, Frohwirth, et al. 2017), creating what legal scholar David Cohen and sociologist Carole Joffe (2020) astutely term an "obstacle course." Notably, this outcome of not being able to obtain a wanted abortion because of policy restrictions on abortion care is not equivalent to choosing to have a baby.

In Maryland, the policy landscape was markedly different. Maryland allowed state public funds to cover abortion care for public insurance recipients; allowed abortion without gestational age restriction through viability and after if the pregnant person's life or health was endangered or there was a fetal anomaly; did not require a waiting period; and did not mandate counseling or ultrasound viewing (Guttmacher Institute 2018b). For these reasons, Maryland is generally understood as an abortion-supportive state in terms of access and availability of care. That did not mean, however, that respondents in Maryland faced no structural obstacles to abortion care.

Despite their divergent policy environments, Louisiana and Maryland share a similar organization of abortion provision—and this organization serves as a potential structural barrier to abortion. Abortion care is marginalized in medicine, mostly taking place in stand-alone outpatient clinics (Jones, Witwer, and Jerman 2019). Although this organization of care holds advantages, including ensuring that patients interact with staff who are not antiabortion, it has also served to silo abortion care delivery: proportionately few abortions are provided in hospitals and physician offices (Jones, Witwer, and Jerman 2019). Additionally, few obstetrician-gynecologists provide abortion care (Grossman, Grindlay, et al. 2019). This is not due to specialization or lack of skill; first-trimester aspiration abortion is equivalent to the procedural treatment for a miscarriage, and ob-gyns regularly perform far more complicated interventions, including surgeries such as cesareans. Nor is it strictly the outcome of individual physicians' preferences around abortion care. Sociologist Lori Freedman (2010) finds that organizational structures and institutional norms conspire to discourage physicians interested in providing abortion care from doing so. Mainstream medicine also regularly fails to facilitate access to abortion care; a substantial minority of physicians who do not provide abortions also decline to refer to abortion care (Desai, Jones, and Castle 2018).

In both Louisiana and Maryland, the marginalization of abortion care in medicine meant that respondents did not expect to obtain abortion care from their regular healthcare providers. Most respondents had already internalized this, speaking of having to "find a clinic" to obtain an abortion. From the outset, in other words, respondents' consideration of abortion was premised on the expectation that they would have to personally find a provider, traversing a different path than that they typically followed to obtain health care.

In Maryland, there were twenty-five abortion clinics during data collection (Jones, Witwer, and Jerman 2019). In Louisiana, it was a different story. In addition to the restrictive abortion laws affecting patient experiences described above, Louisiana had several policies regulating abortion providers. Colloquially known as TRAP laws (Targeted Regulation of Abortion Providers), these laws establish requirements for providers such as that abortion-providing physicians have local hospital admitting privileges or that clinic facilities meet the standards of an ambulatory surgery center. Research has shown no health or safety benefit of admitting privileges laws, but has shown real consequences to pregnant people's access to abortion services if clinicians are unable to secure privileges (Berglas, Battistelli, et al. 2018). Likewise, there is no evidence that obtaining an abortion in an ambulatory surgery center versus an outpatient clinic is safer (S. Roberts, Upadhyay, et al. 2018). These laws do have the clear effect of increasing the costs of running a stand-alone abortion clinic, and the costs of compliance may be overwhelming for some clinics. Physician-researcher Daniel Grossman and colleagues found that a Texas TRAP law led to a substantial decrease in service availability in the state (Grossman, White, et al. 2017). In turn, the limited number of providers can contribute to the inability of some pregnant people to have an abortion (Grossman, White, et al. 2017; Jerman, Frohwirth, et al. 2017), and, for those able to obtain an abortion, to an increase in second-trimester abortions as people have longer waits to see a provider (White et al. 2019). The specific landscape of abortion care in Louisiana was characterized by scarcity: at the start of data collection, there were five abortion-providing facilities in the state; by the end of the two-year data collection, one had closed (Jones, Witwer, and Jerman 2019).

As with the policy-related obstacles to abortion, the inability to overcome obstacles produced by the organization of abortion care neutralizes a decision for abortion, regardless of the reason for abortion. As public health scientist Jenny O'Donnell and colleagues found in interviews conducted in rural Appalachia, an underserved, low-income area, when accessing abortion care is infeasible, pregnant women who do not want to continue their pregnancy may resign themselves to that outcome (O'Donnell, Goldberg, et al. 2018). The logic for this phenomenon is straightforward:

without abortion care as a resource, one cannot implement an abortion decision. Still, it bears stating that women under these circumstances were not continuing their pregnancies because they wanted to have a baby.

Culture

There is, thus, a robust literature supporting the idea that some people do not obtain an abortion after considering one because structural barriers make abortion unchooseable. Structures, however, do not operate alone. They do not come into being alone, they are not reproduced alone, and they do not influence behavior alone. Culture matters. Culture, like structures, can encourage or discourage some lines of action over others. And, like structures, culture varies over time and place and may differentially influence some populations.

Cultural sociologists have a number of theories about culture in action that are of analytical use in making sense of why pregnant people who consider abortion do not obtain one. The word "culture" is used to mean different, often overlapping things. I use "culture" to describe the ever-present, all-encompassing field of discursive and actionable opportunities and constraints in which people act. All individual experiences take place in a social, collective context—that is, culture—that shapes ideas, beliefs, and, ultimately, actions. Attending to culture is an important antidote to the reasons framework, which privileges the individual at the expense of the interpersonal and the social. A cultural approach decenters individualism, understanding that the scope of individual agency is always constrained, and the direction of that agency is channeled by culture.

Abortion has a cogent cultural meaning in the contemporary United States. Legal scholar Carol Sanger (2016, 651) argues that abortion is not just about pregnancy: it is about "medicine, religion, rights, regulation, morality, sex, gender, families, and politics." Rhetorician Nathan Stormer (2015) similarly argues that rates of abortion have been used as political proxies for social issues ranging from autonomy to morality to civilization. While this operation takes place at the level of social discourse, it follows that the social meaning of abortion could have an effect on individual pregnancy decision making.

I focus specifically on the impact of cultural narratives about abortion on respondents' decision making. Narratives are ways of making sense of the meaning of abortion. They convey collective agreement about what abortion means generally as well as who abortion patients are—and they naturalize these meanings, making them appear common sense and even taken for granted. Cultural narratives are sometimes called schemas or frames. The idea is that they are a way of understanding something, often in the absence of personal experience. Narratives may come from religion, family, the media, and popular culture. And they may or may not be grounded in empirical reality. Sociologist Gretchen Sisson and I (2016) show, for example, that the representation of people who have abortions in American film and television deviates from the demographics of actual abortion patients. In particular, pop culture overrepresents young, white, nulliparous abortion patients and underrepresents low-income, already-parenting, and nonwhite abortion patients. To the extent people form their ideas about who gets abortions based on representations they see on television, their beliefs will not match reality. In a review of the sociology of storytelling, sociologist Francesca Polletta and colleagues (2011) argue that narrative does the work of institutions, naturalizing power and inequality. Cultural narratives, in other words, are importantly related to social structures, even as they operate via different mechanisms.

Cultural narratives can shape people's understanding of the meaning of abortion and motivate action—or inaction. In his dual process model of culture in action, sociologist Stephen Vaisey (2009) proposes that culture is internalized and often unarticulated or even unconscious. Once internalized, cultural meanings influence action. Culture is not just something that surrounds us but also something with practical impacts, although these impacts may occur without conscious awareness. Abortion in the United States is not a neutral concept; it is broadly stigmatized (Kimport and

Freedman 2018; Kumar, Hessini, and Mitchell 2009; Norris et al. 2011). Consistent with sociologists Bruce Link and Jo Phelan's (2001) principles of stigma, research shows that abortion providers and patients are socially labeled as different, associated with negative attributes, separated from a presumed "us," and may experience discrimination and status loss because of their association with abortion (see Kimport and Freedman 2018 for a review). This was not always the case. In the nineteenth century, abortion was legal and quietly tolerated (Reagan 1997; Smith-Rosenberg 1986). Historian James Mohr (1979) has shown how the criminalization of abortion and cultural shift from tolerance to vilification was part of a nineteenth-century campaign by physicians to discredit midwives and other competing health practitioners (see also Stormer 2015), illustrating how the cultural meaning of abortion has changed over time. For pregnant people considering abortion in the current cultural moment, the prevalence of abortion stigmatization and anti-abortion cultural narratives may affect their decision making, with the upshot that they consider but do not obtain an abortion.

While research has examined how abortion is framed in social movement activism (Ginsburg 1998; Luker 1984; McCaffrey and Keys 2000; Meyer and Staggenborg 2008; Rohlinger 2002) and public discourse (Rohlinger 2006, 2015), less work has investigated the cultural narratives pregnant people and abortion patients themselves engage with. One exception is sociologist Mallary Allen's (2014) analysis of personal abortion stories posted online. Allen traces the dominant arcs and characteristics of published narratives, noting distinct narrative patterns among online posters who support versus oppose abortion rights. The dominant narratives in support of abortion rights, she argues, are constructed in ways that render them consistent with contemporary middle-class, gendered values. In contrast, the dominant narratives among posters opposed to abortion rights, including those who claim they regret their abortion, allow for more diverse circumstances. Extant cultural narratives may thus be more available to some groups than others in making sense of their own circumstances and abortion decision making.

Other research has documented narratives of the meaning of abortion in poor women's accounts of becoming single mothers. Public policy scholar Kathryn Edin and sociologist Maria Kefalas's (2011) ethnography of poor single mothers in the Philadelphia area finds that some of the women they followed said they rejected abortion for an unexpected pregnancy because they saw choosing abortion as failing to take responsibility for their own actions in becoming pregnant. Edin and Kefalas do not deeply probe participants' consideration (or lack thereof) of abortion, nor do they focus on pregnancy decision making, but they nonetheless offer evidence of the operation of cultural narratives about abortion in their participants' decision to become single mothers.

The women I interviewed may have been unable to place themselves in existing cultural narratives of choosing abortion, particularly to the extent that such narratives do not allow space for people in their circumstances. As with structural barriers to abortion, this inability to envision choosing abortion may mean women continue their pregnancies but does not mean they want to have a baby.

Experience and Embodiment

Distinct but tightly related to both structures and culture, the final way I seek to understand the experiences of women who considered but did not obtain an abortion is through the lens of experience and embodiment. I conceptualize embodiment as the interplay among bodily experience, emotions, perceptions, meaning making, and the self. I posit multiple pathways through which experience and embodiment might matter, centering the historically informed distrust of medicine, itself an effect of racism (Boyd et al. 2020), by some marginalized groups. For one, respondents might consider abortion but not obtain one because of experiential knowledge of abortion. With current estimates that one in four women will have an abortion in her lifetime (Jones and Jerman 2017), this experiential knowledge might inform their current decision making, particularly if there was an aspect of their previous experience with abortion care that was unpleasant, or worse. Reproductive events are both social and corporeal (Van der Sijpt 2014), and abortion can be painful (Bélanger, Melzack, and Lauzon 1989; Penney 2006; Renner et al. 2009). Respondents with previous experience of an abortion may associate the choice with pain or other discomfort and may therefore consider but not obtain an abortion. This is not the same as wanting to have a baby.

Pregnant people who have not had a prior abortion, too, might negatively anticipate what abortion would be like. They might have what I term "anticipated negative embodiment" of abortion based on their general knowledge of abortion and/or bad experiences of health care generally. In both Louisiana and Maryland, to obtain a legal abortion, pregnant people must interact with a healthcare professional. Some populations are better served than others by the healthcare system. In particular, research has shown that people of color receive poorer care than white populations, including in pain management (Hoffman et al. 2016), cancer treatment (Esnaola and Ford 2012), and HIV/AIDS care (Heslin et al. 2005). Scholars have shown that this disparity persists even when income is controlled for (Balasubramanian et al. 2012). Present-day health inequities exist in the legacy of the historical exploitation of communities of color by medicine, including not only the infamous Tuskegee experiment wherein Black men were denied a known treatment for syphilis in order to observe the disease's progression, but also other medical experiments before and since (Gamble 1997; Washington 2006). Indeed, as sociologist Troy Duster (2003) astutely argues, medicine has been conscripted into the reification of racial hierarchies and racism in the United States, deployed as purportedly objective "science" in order to naturalize socially constructed racial inequalities.

Specific to reproductive health care, the medical profession has a history of experimenting on the bodies of women of color (Owens 2017; D. Roberts 1999) and of eugenics (Flavin 2008). And this experimentation has not been restricted to the fringes of medicine. Figures central to the history of medicine are included in this legacy, such as the supposed founder of gynecology, whose breakthroughs were developed through experimentation on the bodies of enslaved Black women (Ojanuga 1993) and exploitation of the same women's medical and intellectual labor (Owens 2017). Their ability to give informed consent was inherently compromised by their enslaved status. Historians have also pointed to the initial testing of the hormonal contraceptive pill with women in Puerto Rico—who were given a dosage substantially higher than the combination currently used, as well as limited information on its mechanism—as an occasion where reproductive medicine exploited women of color (Gordon 2002). Historically, Black and brown women have been sterilized by the state and by paternalistic doctors without their consent (Nelson 2003; Schoen 2005; Stern 2005).

These practices of controlling the reproduction of particular populations extend into the contemporary moment. Incarcerated women in the state of California were sterilized without their consent as recently as 2010 (Roth and Ainsworth 2015). Socially marginalized populations, including low-income women and women who use drugs, have been coerced in recent decades by state programs into using long-acting contraceptive methods in exchange for basic services (Boonstra et al. 2000; M. Morgan 2004). And pregnancy and birth outcomes are still marked by race disparities, with white women having better outcomes than Black women in regard to infant mortality and maternal mortality (Anachebe and Sutton 2003). Between 2011 and 2016 in Louisiana, which already had a higher maternal mortality rate than the nation as a whole, Black women were four times more likely to experience a pregnancy-related death than white women (Kieltyka et al. 2018). Maryland, too, had a higher maternal mortality rate than the United States as a whole between 2010 and 2014, and Black women's maternal mortality rate was two and a half times greater than white women's (Maryland Department of Health and Mental Hygiene 2017). These epidemiological findings come from and perpetuate the lived reality of racism. As anthropologist Khiara Bridges (2011) argues, the *process* of reproduction—including the way health care and patient care are organized—itself reproduces race and racial inequality.

Socially disadvantaged people recognize and feel these racial inequities in health care. As public health scientist Thomas LaVeist and colleagues persuasively document, socially disadvantaged groups report experiencing more discrimination in health care settings than their advantaged counterparts: women (compared to men), people of color (compared to whites), and low-income people (compared to higher-income people) perceive greater discrimination from healthcare system workers (LaVeist, Rolley, and Diala 2003). Evidence of perceived discrimination is found in reproductive healthcare settings in specific. Public health scholars Sheryl Thorburn and Laura Bogart (2005) found that 67 percent of the Black women they surveyed who had visited a healthcare practitioner for family planning care reported experiencing race-based discrimination. These experiences and knowledge of others' experiences of discrimination can lead to medical mistrust and healthcare avoidance, with individuals intentionally opting out of using the healthcare system out of a desire to avoid experiencing discrimination (Boyd et al. 2020; D'Anna et al. 2018; LaVeist, Isaac, and Williams 2009). This could be at play for some respondents. Avoidance of health care by low-income or poor Black women, even for a wanted abortion, could contribute to considering but not obtaining an abortion.

Plan of the Book

In this book, I trace how respondents made sense of their pregnancies, their pregnancy options or lack thereof, and their reproductive agency by attending to the way that these three factors could render abortion unchooseable. These women's circumstances were conditioned and constrained by state-level policy, the organization and availability of abortion care, cultural narratives about abortion, their own experiences of health care, and their gendered, raced, and classed social location. This book examines how power and inequality make it difficult for specific groups of people to enact their reproductive goals and achieve reproductive autonomy, how they can end up with no real choice. I apply an intersectional perspective in my analysis, attending to how race and class disadvantage not only constrained the lives of the women I interviewed but also magnified the power of the structural and cultural obstacles to reproductive autonomy they faced.

I should clarify here that I do not believe that all respondents would have chosen abortion had it been a real choice for them. Nor do I take any position on what pregnancy outcome would be best for them; that is something only they, with important others in their lives, can determine. What my analysis reveals, nonetheless, is how abortion was rendered unchooseable for them. This inhibited their reproductive autonomy to make a pregnancy decision, whether to terminate or continue the pregnancy. That is, in not being able to choose abortion, they were likewise constrained in their ability to choose the circumstances under which they wanted to have a baby. What I am interested in unpacking, then, is not the fact that these women did not have abortions but, instead, how structures, culture, and expectations of what the experience of abortion would be like impeded their ability to determine whether and under what circumstances they wanted to have a baby. In this way, my work is informed by a reproductive justice framework, a firmly intersectional perspective developed by women of color activists that holds that people have the right to have a child, to not have a child, and to raise the children they have in safe and sustainable communities (Ross, Derkas, et al. 2017).

My analysis begins in chapter 2, with an examination of how structural obstacles became barriers to abortion for respondents in both Louisiana and Maryland. For the most part, these barriers were the result of restrictive state policies on abortion, but they also owed to features of the landscape of abortion care provision and entrenched structural inequalities of race and class. Because of these structural barriers, including barriers not ostensibly related to abortion, these women were unable to obtain an abortion, rendering their pregnancy "choice" moot. In practice, abortion was unchooseable. I close the chapter with discussion of three women who sought to work around the structural obstacles they faced by attempting to end their pregnancies on their own, outside of a clinical setting. By examining their (failed) efforts, I show both their agentic efforts in the face of potent structural barriers and the insurmountability of those barriers.

In chapters 3 and 4, I identify the pervasive cultural narratives about abortion in respondents' lives and unpack their origins, detailing their association with the antiabortion movement. Chapter 3 focuses on narratives about the fetus, chapter 4 on narratives about the pregnant person. I describe how these resonant narratives affected respondents' decision making. Specifically, I argue that these narratives determined what it meant for these respondents to choose abortion, supplying meanings that conflicted with respondents' sense of themselves as moral, responsible people. With such meanings for choosing abortion, abortion became unchooseable, even as most continued to feel no attachment to their ongoing pregnancy. I show that because women like these respondents are more likely to have an unexpected pregnancy—itself an effect of inequality—they are also more likely to have to navigate narratives that curtail their ability to choose abortion.

In chapter 5, I examine the effect of experience and embodiment on respondents' pregnancy decision making. Whether because of personal experience of abortion, exposure to unsatisfactory providers, or experiences of medical mistreatment, some of the women I interviewed anticipated that the experience of abortion would be negative—or worse. They did not want to have the embodied experience of abortion (again), and this informed their decision not to seek an abortion. At the end of this chapter, I discuss the experiences of three women, different from those in chapter 2, who also attempted and failed to end their pregnancy on their own. Their accounts illustrate a distinction between wanting an abortion and wanting a clinic-based abortion.

Throughout these four substantive chapters, I underscore three key findings: First, abortion was unchooseable for most respondents despite being legal and, in theory, available. It was unchooseable in various ways, as the chapters delineate, but the collective takeaway is that some pregnant people in the United States cannot choose abortion because structural and cultural forces have made it impossible to choose, which means they have no real choice in their pregnancy outcome. Second, the social location of the women I interviewed made them specifically vulnerable to factors producing abortion as unchooseable. The inequality they experienced from their low-income status and, for most of the respondents, Black racial identity was central to how abortion became unchooseable for them. Abortion may be unchooseable for other populations as well, but its production for these women was an effect of extant race, class, and gender inequality.

Third, these chapters illustrate the breadth and depth of antiabortion frameworks in contemporary U.S. society. The operation of the constraints against choosing abortion I enumerate exceeds the site of abortion care delivery. Policy restrictions, the organization of abortion care, antiabortion cultural narratives, and anticipated negative embodiment of abortion made abortion unchooseable even among those who had no contact with abortion care providers. For a full understanding of how antiabortion frameworks have polluted pregnancy decision making—and how and for whom there is no real pregnancy choice—we must look beyond the pregnant people who present for abortion care. That said, the antiabortion movement is not the sole contributor to the denial of reproductive autonomy. Medical racism and poverty, sometimes in combination with antiabortion movement actions and narratives, are also clear contributors to abortion being unchooseable and some women having no real choice.

Finally, in chapter 6, I draw on the accounts of a small subset of respondents who considered abortion but did not obtain one because they wanted to have a baby. They did not, in other words, continue their pregnancies expressly because abortion was unchooseable but, instead, because they chose to. While some women in the earlier chapters did come to feel positively about continuing their pregnancy, this was an adaptation after discovering that abortion was unchooseable. The women in this chapter, in contrast, felt positively about their pregnancy at the time they ruled out abortion. It was why they did not choose abortion. Nonetheless, I find evidence of constraints on their reproductive agency as well.

In summarizing their decision making—and unlike in their nuanced accounts of their decision making—they drew on the same antiabortion cultural narratives that rendered abortion unchooseable for other respondents to justify their pregnancy outcome. In a discursive landscape wherein the desire of low-income women and women of color to parent is questioned, discouraged, or obstructed, deploying antiabortion cultural narratives to explain continuation of pregnancy can be a strategy to deflect racist and classed challenges of these women's right to parent. Their experiences illustrate not only a strategic deployment of hegemonic antiabortion cultural narratives to discursively account for pregnancy outcomes but also the dearth of narratives affirming marginalized populations' right to parent. They seemingly had a choice, but no socially accepted narratives for centering their desire to parent in their own storytelling.

I close the book with a summary of my argument that structures (including structures not ostensibly related to abortion), cultural narratives, and anticipation of a negative embodied experience of abortion—all of which rest on and/or are magnified by extant race and class inequality—can render abortion unchooseable, denying women reproductive autonomy in pregnancy decision making. I discuss the role of the antiabortion movement in these processes, including how its efforts leverage existing inequalities. Finally, I offer some ideas about what would make true pregnancy choice of whether and when to parent real for all pregnant people.

Conclusion

Before turning to the substantive chapters, it is important to point out that there are few white voices in this book, and one of them is mine. As the book's author, it is a big one. I am financially stable and have completed a graduate education, two characteristics that also differentiate me from the women I interviewed. I discuss some of the implications of these differences for data collection in the Methodological Appendix. Here, though, I want to discuss how my social location matters for this analysis. I do not have experiential access to the cultural, racial, socioeconomic, and educational contextual components that may have been at play in respondents' decision making. During both interviewing and analysis, I most certainly missed digging deeper into elements of respondents' lives that matter for understanding their experience of considering and not obtaining an abortion. Respondents themselves may have chosen not to share aspects of their experiences and personalities that they preferred to keep private from me or thought I would misunderstand or judge negatively. What I can offer is a partial, situated knowledge (Haraway 1988) that is conditioned by the differences between my social location and those of respondents, and transparency about the social locations from which that knowledge emerges.

In this book's analyses, I have sought to be radically reflexive of my racial and socioeconomic social location, starting from a place of empathy, respect, and deference. The women in this book are experts on their own lives. Their accounts make sense. Their choices deserve respect. They have been subject to offensively unequal structures, policies, racism, classism, and sexism. This book endeavors to give voice to people who have historically been silenced or, when heard, listened to with suspicion and in comparison to a norm that is white and class-privileged. This book insists on the scholarly and social importance of their voices. These women's accounts tell us about where we are, why we remain here, and at what cost.

2

Policies, Poverty, and
the Organization of Abortion Care

Jayla, a twenty-one-year-old Black woman in Louisiana, discovered she was pregnant at ten weeks gestation, although she did not know she was that far into pregnancy at the time. She was living in unstable housing with her three-year-old, drinking heavily, and using drugs frequently. She did not have the money to pay for an abortion, as she would be required to in Louisiana, but knew it was the right choice for her. She asked her mother for financial help. Her mother was initially reluctant, asking her to "think about it [more]." Her mother's insistence that Jayla reconsider her desire to obtain an abortion did not change Jayla's thinking about abortion, she explained, "because I still wanted an abortion." It did take time, though. As Jayla related, "She kind of wanted me to, like, I guess dwell on it and think about it. But when I called her [several days later] and I was determined that this is what I want to do, it took her like a few days, and then she just called me out of the blue and was like '[Jayla], I'll give you money if that's what you want to do.'" Even after agreeing to give her daughter the money to pay for an abortion, Jayla's mother, herself financially struggling, needed time to come up with the money.

As Jayla detailed, the time it took her mother to secure the funds for an abortion pushed her past the gestational limit of the nearest clinic: "When my mom finally got enough money for the abortion, that's when my mom called them, and they told my mom that eighteen weeks was the cutoff limit." This was new information to Jayla. Although the facility's eighteen-week limit was below the state's gestational limit, for Jayla it was the de facto limit: she did not know where else to go. She thought she was close to eighteen weeks and feared spending the money to get a sonogram for gestational dating at the abortion clinic only to be told she was over their limit. She searched for a place that would offer her an ultrasound for free, finding a local antiabortion pregnancy resource center that offered free sonograms. Antiabortion pregnancy resource centers are nonprofit, usually evangelical Christian organizations with a mission to dissuade pregnant people from choosing abortion (see also Kimport 2019). There, Jayla received an ultrasound and learned that she was eighteen weeks, two days pregnant. With this information, she understood that abortion was no longer an option for her: "I kind of prepared myself. Almost like took a deep breath, like you know, 'So, I'm about to have another baby.'" Jayla's experience illustrates how structural obstacles to abortion, sometimes in concert with opposition to abortion from loved ones, can stymie women's ability to have an abortion. When Jayla could not implement an abortion decision in practice, her autonomy to choose abortion was likewise eliminated: one cannot choose what one cannot implement.

Jayla's experience of these barriers to abortion was common across the women I interviewed, although the specifics were unique. And although Maryland did not have the same spate of restrictive policies as Louisiana, women in Maryland nonetheless also experienced structural barriers to choosing abortion. In this chapter, I discuss the experiences of respondents who encountered insurmountable structural obstacles to abortion and for whom, because of these barriers, abortion was unchooseable.

Structural Barriers to Abortion

As in Jayla's experience, structural barriers to abortion, including restrictive policies and the organization of abortion care provision, had discernible impacts on many of the Louisiana respondents' experiences of pregnancy decision making, constraining their ability to choose abortion. Michelle, a thirty-six-year-old white woman in Louisiana, faced substantial economic challenges to choosing abortion. She knew from her prior abortion experiences that abortion was expensive without ever calling a clinic. Homeless for the past six months after being kicked out of an in-patient alcohol and drug rehabilitation program because of a relapse, Michelle was financially destitute. She could not afford the $3 copay for medication to manage her diagnosed mental health disorder. She felt, in a word, "hopeless." After Michelle was asked to leave the rehab program, her parents, who had given her money for her previous abortions, ceased communication with her, refusing to respond to her voicemails and texts.

This pregnancy was unexpected. She had a boyfriend who also lived on the streets who helped her feel safe, but she found him controlling and wanted to leave the relationship. She explained: "He's not the right person for me. I just—I got involved with him when I got on the street, and now I'm kind of stuck. . . . He's just very controlling and very jealous for no reason. I think he has— it's becoming more clear he has some psychological issues." Michelle never wanted to have children and did not want to continue this pregnancy. Yet she realized that, in practice, abortion was not an option for her. She simply could not afford the out-of-pocket cost of an abortion.

The inability to pay for an abortion was determinative of Michelle's pregnancy outcome. As she summed it up: "If I could have afforded it, I would have had it done right when I found out." As it was, she recognized quite quickly how her financial situation rendered abortion impossible for her to obtain. So she gave up on it without even contacting a clinic. Michelle, in other words, had no choice about whether to continue or terminate her pregnancy. She could not afford an abortion, which eliminated abortion as an outcome for her. This did not mean she felt good about continuing her pregnancy. In fact, struggling to manage her alcohol and drug use, her controlling relationship, her mental illness, and homelessness, she had not paid much attention to her pregnancy at all.

The prohibition on public insurance coverage of abortion was not the only policy that changed the terms of respondents' decision making. Other policy-related factors, such as Louisiana's two-visit requirement, could likewise make choosing abortion impossible. That was the case with Tyler. Tyler, a twenty-six-year-old Black woman in Louisiana, had enough money to pay for a first-trimester procedure. Her work schedule, however, made it difficult to take enough time off to accommodate the state-mandated two-visit requirement. Tyler's employment in an hourly wage job, common for the respondents who were employed, represented inflexible employment. Her parenting responsibilities for her six- and ten-year-old children further constrained her time. By the time she was able to get multiple days off from work, she was in the second trimester of pregnancy and unable to afford the increased out-of-pocket costs for a second-trimester procedure. State policies like the two-visit requirement are likely to disproportionately negatively impact low-income pregnant people like Tyler who have little autonomy over their work schedules. As she elaborated, capturing the limits of the language of "choice" to describe her experience, "women don't really have a choice here [in Louisiana]. I mean, they do, but they make it so hard to make that choice that you really don't have one."

Ultimately, for women like Michelle and Tyler, policies restricting abortion went from an obstacle to navigate to an insurmountable barrier, negating their ability to choose abortion and resulting in their passive decision to continue the pregnancy. Consistent with the research summarized in chapter 1, policy regulation of abortion can make abortion unavailable for some pregnant people. What Michelle's and Tyler's experiences illustrate, further, is how these policies can constrain pregnancy decision making without either woman ever contacting an abortion clinic. While most research has focused on women who present for abortion care, the accounts of these two women suggest that the impact of restrictive policy may be greater than currently measured.

It is also important to make explicit how these policies and institutional structures became consequential. They mattered because of respondents' pre-existing financial circumstances: they were low income or poor. To the extent that reliance on public insurance and the fact that Louisiana bans public insurance coverage of abortion mattered in respondents' inability to choose abortion, this is a specifically classed problem. Whereas more affluent women are likely to have access to money to pay for abortion on their own and, potentially, the social networks and money to get to a provider who is farther away, this is less likely to be true for low-income and poor women. Similarly, people with more class privilege have greater flexibility to miss work or control their work schedules than did women like Tyler.

Poverty, and class more generally, are not independent of the history of race and ongoing racism in the United States. The legacy of slavery, Jim Crow laws, and redlining has largely prevented Black Americans from building wealth (Baradaran 2017; Oliver and Shapiro 2006). Black Americans also have less access to occupational opportunity and, for those who are employed, are regularly paid less than whites in related jobs (Branch and Jackson 2020), contributing to patterns of limited class mobility (Laurison, Dow, and Chernoff 2020). Meanwhile, the ongoing production of financial disadvantage through eviction (Desmond 2016) and mass incarceration (Alexander 2020), practices that disproportionately affect Black Americans, perpetuates the intersection of poverty and Blackness. Most of the respondents found themselves at this intersection. They were thus subject not only to restrictive policies on abortion that were of greater consequence because they were poor, but also to racist policies and practices that produced and cemented that very financial vulnerability. In the lives of low-income and poor Black women, policies regulating abortion work in concert with other policies—often policies not ostensibly related to abortion or reproductive health—to significantly affect their ability to choose abortion.

Other respondents in Louisiana faced obstacles of scarcity that were not about money. Several reported that they were wholly unable to find an abortion provider despite extensive searching. For example, Camille, a thirty-three-year-old Black woman in Louisiana, could not find a local abortion clinic. She began by searching online. After calling two or three of the numbers from the results of her online search of "abortion clinics" and, perplexingly to Camille, reaching locations in Texas and California that would not give her information about obtaining an abortion, one place she called gave her the phone number for a clinic in her area. She called that number and told them, "I'm thinking of going to a place for abortion." In response, Camille related, the receptionist there said, "'Well, we are not an abortion clinic, but we do offer classes. You qualify for your first visit, but you have to pay after that. [Other places charge] between $75 and $100. We offer these classes free.'" Camille figured this was reasonable. She said of the service, "It's like a conversation you have to go through before you get an abortion. And I guess after you complete it, they give you like a form to have to be able to—you don't have to pay [at the abortion clinic]."

When Camille arrived for her appointment, however, she discovered that this place was not what she expected. For one, it was, she said, "totally antiabortion. They won't condone it or send you to one. You end up talking to, like, a crisis counselor for pregnant women and stuff like that." Camille was already ashamed of considering abortion in the first place, fearing the judgment of her family and community. Her conversations at what turned out to be an antiabortion pregnancy resource center contributed to her thinking abortion was not a good pregnancy choice (see also Kimport 2019, 2020). Nonetheless, she explained, had it been easier—or even possible—to find an abortion provider, "I probably would have [had an abortion]. To be honest with you, I probably would have. And I would have just probably talked to God and dealt with it and not told anybody. It would have been something that I dealt with. But it wasn't easy [to find a provider]." For Camille, the inability to find a provider was a primary reason why she did not obtain an abortion after considering it. The entire state of Louisiana had only four abortion clinics by the end of the data collection, meaning that 72 percent of women in Louisiana lived in a county with no abortion clinic (Jones, Witwer, and Jerman 2019). There were not, in other words, many providers for respondents like Camille to find.

Structural Barriers in the Absence of Antiabortion Policies

Although Maryland had none of the restrictions these four Louisiana respondents described and had comparatively high service availability with multiple local abortion providers, some of the Maryland respondents described facing structural barriers to abortion that were strikingly similar to those of their Louisiana counterparts. Their experiences underscore the importance of underlying class and race inequalities and policies ostensibly unrelated to abortion in pregnant people's ability to choose abortion. To the extent that some restrictive policies on abortion gain power over pregnant people's ability to choose abortion by leveraging existing inequalities, as was often the case in Louisiana, these Maryland respondents' accounts demonstrate the potency of non-abortion-related policies and the inequalities they produce to themselves operate as barriers to abortion.

For example, Desiree, a thirty-year-old Black woman in Maryland, had Medicaid insurance but, due to a paperwork error, had lost her coverage right before she discovered her pregnancy. Desiree did not want to be pregnant. She was living in unsafe and poor-quality housing with her four children, actively trying to move to a different, safer neighborhood. Moreover, she had a history of miscarriage, stillbirth, preterm birth, and bleeding during pregnancy, which led her doctors to recommend after her last birth that she never get pregnant again. She was navigating clinical depression and self-medicating with opioids. When she discovered she was pregnant, she was certain she did not want to continue the pregnancy. She scheduled an abortion right away.

Then came the letter telling her that her Medicaid had been cut off at the end of the prior month. Unable to pay her utility bills, Desiree found herself in a financial situation similar to that of the respondents from Louisiana described above. And like those

Louisiana respondents, without her Medicaid, Desiree had to pay for abortion out of pocket. Desiree did not have the money for an abortion. By the time she got her Medicaid reinstated at the end of the following month, her advanced gestation, coupled with her pregnancy history, meant that there were a limited number of providers who could safely care for her. She found a hospital that would perform abortion at her gestation and take her insurance, but they only offered abortion care infrequently, and she would have to wait several weeks for an appointment. Desiree felt at this stage, "What's the point?," since she would be, by then, more than halfway through the typical forty weeks of pregnancy.

In Desiree's case, just as with the women from Louisiana, it was not just the absence of insurance coverage for abortion that mattered for her decision making. Her financial vulnerability also mattered. Other respondents from Maryland underscored how the reality of poverty itself was a structural barrier to abortion. For instance, Khadijah's youngest child was nine years old when Khadijah, a twenty-nine-year-old Black woman in Maryland, discovered this pregnancy. It took her a while to recognize the pregnancy, as her menstrual cycle had never been regular. Moreover, with so many years since her last pregnancy, Khadijah thought perhaps she could no longer get pregnant, attributing the nausea of what turned out to be early pregnancy to something she had eaten. When she learned she was pregnant, at nearly three and a half months' gestation, she and her partner "both decided that it wasn't the right time." She made an appointment for an abortion, sharing her plan with her grandmother, mother, and best friend, all of whom were supportive and understanding.

At the appointment, she disclosed her history of cesareans, prompting the clinic to request she first get a full sonogram at the hospital, as Khadijah understood it, "to make sure I had no scar tissue or anything." It took a week for Khadijah to get an appointment for a sonogram. While she was there, the hospital did a blood test and determined that her iron count was low. Between her low iron and history of cesareans, the physician at the clinic declined to provide an abortion for her "because [she] was a high risk" and provided her with a list of three other providers who could safely care for her. She contacted one of the providers on this list and made an appointment. They told her there was a waiting list, which confused her: "I've never known for an abortion clinic to put you on a waiting list." A week and a half later, they called her and told her they had an immediate opening and that she needed to be at the facility within thirty minutes. Khadijah could not manage that timing: "I have no car, so I had to depend on somebody else," such as her grandmother, who needed at least a day's notice in order to drive her. The bus would have taken longer than thirty minutes and, besides, "I didn't have no money at the time to catch the bus."

Khadijah could not make it to that appointment because she was poor, a circumstance that was consequential because of her high-risk status. If Khadijah had access to transportation—even enough money for a taxi—she could have obtained the abortion. As it was, although the provider offered to continue to keep her on the waiting list, she felt it was not worth it. She did not see how she could make it next time if the call came. While the scholarly literature on fatalism, wherein lack of proactive health behaviors is interpreted as evidence that individuals doubt their ability to affect a health outcome, might explain Khadijah's behavior under this rubric, such an analysis underappreciates the quantity of effort Khadijah did undertake. As with other research on health activities among socially marginalized communities (e.g., Drew and Schoenberg 2011), Khadijah's assessment that further action would be futile occurred only after experiencing inadequate healthcare access and scheduling practices she found suspect (which I discuss further in chapter 5). In our interview, she noted that she never changed her mind about wanting an abortion, even as abortion was not something she was practically able to choose. She said of her partner and herself, "We had already made the decision. And yes, the decision was already made. It just didn't work out the way I wanted it."

In Maryland, as in Louisiana, respondents did not expect to receive referrals or have their regular healthcare provider facilitate their entry to abortion care. Even as Maryland respondents had a greater field of abortion providers available to them, with twenty-five clinics in the state operating at the start of data collection, the onus of navigating obtaining care was on the respondent. This was distinct from prenatal care in both states, access to which was readily facilitated by other healthcare providers (S. Roberts, Wingo, and Kimport 2020). For respondents like Claudine, a twenty-four-year-old Black woman in Maryland who sought deep sedation for her abortion, facilitating her own access to abortion meant calling multiple clinics. While abortion clinics commonly offer oral medications or moderate sedation for a first-trimester aspiration abortion, deep sedation requires different safety protocols, so it is not offered at all clinics. This is what Claudine found as she searched. She related, "I guess there was nothing like that [deep sedation], because I had to be woke through the whole thing. So, I kept trying to call different places. And months kept going by and kept going by." When she finally found a clinic that offered deep sedation, they had no available appointments. She found another clinic and made an appointment, only to discover when she arrived that they did not, in fact, offer deep sedation. During this time, her gestation had advanced, and she learned she would have to travel farther away to obtain an abortion. Claudine did not have a car, rendering abortion no longer a possibility. In effect, the structure of abortion care provision—that it was not facilitated by regular healthcare providers—combined with her poverty and associated lack of access to transportation eliminated Claudine's ability to obtain the kind of care she wanted. Resigned, she said, "There's nothing I can do about it."

What these Maryland-based experiences illustrate is the ubiquity of poverty in obstructing these women's ability to choose abortion. They faced structural barriers to choosing abortion rooted in the organization of abortion care provision and entrenched, racialized poverty. Their accounts expose the baseline features consistent across respondents in both Louisiana and Maryland: poverty and the marginalization of abortion care. While there is clear evidence that Louisiana's policy environment has exacerbated the consequences of poverty and the organization of abortion care for many pregnant people in the state, the experiences of Maryland respondents show how policies and practices that do not intend to restrict abortion can nonetheless make abortion impossible to choose. And the populations these policies and practices affect are specific: low-income and poor women and women of color. Still, although structural barriers did render abortion unchooseable for some Maryland respondents, such barriers to abortion were more common in Louisiana than in Maryland. In analyses of quantitative data collected at the same recruitment sites, Sarah Roberts and colleagues found that pregnant women entering prenatal care in Louisiana who reported considering but not obtaining an abortion were more likely than their counterparts in Maryland to report a policy-related barrier to abortion (S. Roberts, Kimport, et al. 2019).

Others' Opposition to Abortion

For some respondents in both Louisiana and Maryland, structural obstacles to abortion were consequential because of opposition to abortion from important others in their lives. After all, one way to overcome structural obstacles is with financial and instrumental support from others. For some of the women I interviewed, as with Jayla from the beginning of the chapter, opposition to abortion from others impeded their ability to successfully leverage their social networks to pay for abortion and find an abortion provider.

This was true for Mercedes, a twenty-three-year-old Hispanic woman in Louisiana. Mercedes was scared when she discovered she was pregnant. She did not want to be pregnant. She called her mother. As Mercedes expected, her mother was very disappointed, having hoped that Mercedes would go to college and get married before becoming pregnant. Mercedes described the phone call: "She [my mother] was like, 'Well, I'm going to pay for your abortion.'" Mercedes told her boyfriend, and they were "leaning towards abortion, because my mom said she was going to pay for it." While Mercedes's mother's encouragement for choosing abortion surely influenced her thinking, Mercedes's ability to choose abortion was pointedly contingent on securing funding. That promise of funding soon disappeared, however, as her mother's personal opposition to abortion overtook her desire to support Mercedes. Mercedes explained, "I called her weeks later, after my [first] appointment, and she's like, 'Well, I'm not going to give you money for it. It's a sin, and I hope—I wish you and the baby a healthy life.' And like, she just hung up on me."

Without her mother's financial support, Mercedes and her boyfriend realized that paying for an abortion was prohibitively difficult. The effort she anticipated having to undertake to find the money did not seem worth it, and she and her boyfriend began preparing for a baby. In Mercedes's case, as for several other respondents, opposition to abortion by loved ones had consequential power in their ability to choose abortion—a power it would not have if abortion were covered by public insurance.

Opposition to abortion from loved ones also mattered for respondents' ability to find an abortion provider, which itself could have consequences for choosing abortion. For example, LaToya, a twenty-three-year-old Black woman in Louisiana, experienced difficulty finding a provider because of opposition to abortion from her mother. LaToya had not expected or wanted to be pregnant: her relationship to the man involved was casual. As she spent more time with him, it became clearer to her that she did not want the relationship to grow. She explained, "The more I learned about him, the more I wasn't really attracted to him." LaToya was having regular periods, and they had used condoms when they had sex, so she never imagined she could be pregnant. She let their relationship fade into nonexistence. She said, "I felt like I wasn't going to be able to deal with [him] and couldn't really change [him] because that's who he was. . . . We just stopped talking, and I didn't bother to, you know, talk to him anymore or find him." When she asked around about him weeks later, she learned that he had moved away.

A few months later, she went to the doctor because she was having headaches and unexplained vomiting. They gave her a pregnancy test that came out positive. Deeply in shock, LaToya left the doctor without finding out how far into pregnancy she was. She explained, "I went home. I didn't really do anything after that. I just remember going home. I don't think I ate anything. I cried a little. Then I think I just went to sleep." Unable to cope with the pregnancy, LaToya ignored it, kept to herself, and focused on her work: "I was really in denial for a long time." LaToya did not tell anyone about her pregnancy for two months. Geographically isolated from family, with few local friends, and financially unstable, she despaired about being pregnant.

LaToya did not want to continue this pregnancy. She had no idea how to find an abortion provider, though, and asked her mother for help. Her mother was explicit that she would not help LaToya because of her opposition to abortion. LaToya explained, "She didn't really tell me what to do because she didn't agree with me. So, she just told me to make sure I was ready if that's what I wanted to do. She didn't really give me information on how to have an abortion or who to call or nothing like that." Eventually, LaToya's cousin told her about a local abortion clinic. When she presented for care at the abortion clinic, she was nearly at the state's gestational limit for abortion. She had no idea she was so far along: "I thought I was something lower." She continued, "They told me that I was really far along in my pregnancy. And it was basically now or never." The marginalization of abortion care and her mother's opposition to abortion, alongside her own denial, contributed to LaToya's delayed presentation for abortion care.

Her delayed presentation for care, in turn, meant the abortion would be more expensive, as the cost of abortion increases with gestation. LaToya had the funds to pay for a second-trimester abortion in her bank account. The dilemma was accessing those funds. LaToya did not have enough time to withdraw the money before she passed the state's gestational limit, and the clinic required full payment in cash. She summed up, "Then it was the weekend. And then they were like, it was going to be $2,600. And I couldn't get all that money together in time." To the extent that the marginalization of abortion care in medicine and the regulation of abortion providers contributed to the small number of clinics in the area and associated lack of choice among providers, LaToya had no alternative to this cash-only policy. And the state's regulation of abortion care meant she had to pay out of pocket for abortion care and was subject to a gestational limit. The clinic, for its part, may have implemented a cash-only policy in an effort to keep costs down by not paying credit card processing fees. This is to say, the policy itself was not designed to make it difficult for LaToya to have an abortion, even if that was its effect. Ultimately, LaToya's experience was constrained by several structural barriers, including the ban on public insurance coverage of abortion, the marginalization of abortion care, and the subsequent associated limited number of available providers, as well as the clinic's payment policy.

As LaToya left the clinic that day, knowing she would not return, an antiabortion protester handed her a flyer about adoption. Explaining what made her decide not to obtain an abortion, she said, "All of it—the cost, the flyer, my mother and everything." After leaving the clinic, LaToya waited more than two months before entering prenatal care at thirty-one weeks into her pregnancy. She was not attached to her pregnancy. Even as people in her life insisted that she would love her baby once it was born, LaToya was doubtful. When I interviewed her, she was eight months pregnant, and she said, "I still don't feel like—I just don't feel like it's for me. I still don't feel like I'm going to be in love with my baby. Now that I'm a little more open with it [the pregnancy], some friend had said to me, he told me, 'Once you give birth, it'll change.' But as of right now I don't feel it changing at all, and I'm due any day now." When I spoke with her, LaToya was sad and lonely. She regularly stopped during the interview to cry quietly and was vocally appreciative of getting the opportunity— the first opportunity she had had so far, she said—to talk about her experience. LaToya was bereft that she was continuing her pregnancy and, despite trying her best to have an abortion, had been structurally prevented from doing so. This was not having reproductive autonomy.

Opposition to abortion from loved ones magnified the effect of structural barriers to abortion for respondents in Maryland as well. Although Maryland does cover abortion care through public insurance, there are a few loopholes in this coverage. The insurance Mariah, a twenty-five-year-old Black woman in Maryland, had fell through one of those loopholes. In practice, her circumstances were thus similar to those of low-income respondents in Louisiana and other states that ban public insurance coverage of abortion. There were other complications in Mariah's life. Mariah was in an abusive marriage. Her husband was physically and verbally abusive when they first got together and had continued to be since they married a year before our interview. Although many of her friends and family knew her husband was violent toward her, Mariah felt they were reasonably unsympathetic because she had stayed with him and married him. Experiencing violence, though, was not new to Mariah. Her mother abused her as a child, the father of her oldest son was physically and emotionally abusive, and she became pregnant with her oldest daughter from a sexual assault. Mariah did not want to be abused but also did not know how to make things different. Reporting the abuse, she anticipated, would remove her from her children—and then who would care for them?

When Mariah first thought she might be pregnant, she, her husband, and her four children were homeless. Her youngest child was less than a year old, and the pregnancy had been dangerous for her health. She explained to her husband, "If I am pregnant, I don't want to have a baby." She told me that she elaborated on why, citing the state of their relationship, telling her husband, "We're not financially in the right place. We're not emotionally or mentally in the right place. You and I as a whole aren't in the right place." Her husband agreed that, were she pregnant, abortion would be the right choice for them.

Once Mariah took a pregnancy test and it came out positive, however, her husband changed his mind. He rescinded support for choosing abortion: "When we found out I was pregnant, he wanted the baby. There was nothing I could say about it." Mariah felt devastated and blamed herself. She said, "I was upset at the fact that, damn, I did it again. I'm stuck again. And then already pregnancy's just hard on my body. And I'm like, damn, I'm setting myself up again for a hard-ass pregnancy with a man who could care less, give two shits about me." Even with her husband's opposition, Mariah still wanted an abortion. She shared her feelings with a friend who agreed that the pregnancy was not a good thing but would not help Mariah obtain an abortion. As Mariah explained, "She's not going to help me do it . . . because I did it to myself."

She looked into abortion on her own. Mariah had no financial resources, her husband and friend refused to help her, and she was battling her own deep feelings of depression and low self-worth. She called several clinics for prices and then her insurance to find out about coverage for abortion, learning from a Medicaid representative that her kind of public insurance covered abortion only in certain exceptional circumstances. Understanding she would have to pay for an abortion out of pocket, Mariah gave up on pursuing one. She said, "I'm forced to have the baby."

Ideational Impacts

Opposition to abortion by important others could amplify the effect of structural obstacles in other ways as well. For some Louisiana respondents, like Paige, a thirty-one-year-old Black woman, opposition to abortion from friends and family combined with structural obstacles to affect their motivation to overcome structural barriers to abortion—and thus their ability to choose abortion. Paige did not expect to become pregnant. She and her boyfriend had been together just under six months and had been having relationship problems. Paige was not sure they would stay together. She wanted to focus on finding a job, establishing a career, and offering stability to her two sons, ages eight and ten. The prospect of "starting over" with a baby was daunting, as Paige felt she had already sacrificed her own employment aspirations in order to care for her two sons when they were young. When she got a positive result on a store-bought pregnancy test, Paige was "undecided" about continuing her pregnancy. After a difficult week of Paige and her boyfriend working through this information, her boyfriend abdicated responsibility for the pregnancy decision, "just saying it's up to me, whatever I wanted to do." Paige kept going "back and forth" about her desired pregnancy outcome, eventually deciding abortion was the right decision for her. In choosing to seek an abortion, she was alone; the select family members she told about her pregnancy all encouraged her to continue it.

Once Paige found a clinic to call, the staffer she spoke with explained the pricing system, and Paige realized that obtaining an abortion would be even more difficult than she had imagined. She did not have the money. She asked her boyfriend for money, and he had nothing to offer. She estimated that were she to try "extra, extra, extra hard," she might be able to raise about $200, which was not enough to cover the cost of an abortion. After about a month, Paige "started to feel bad about if [she] was to get rid of it." Her family's support for continuing the pregnancy and opposition to abortion weighed on her mind, making the idea of working hard to find the money to pay for an abortion more difficult to fathom. Combined with the perceived immense out-of-pocket cost of abortion, Paige felt like there were "two things against it": the cost of abortion and the idea of working to overcome the cost barrier for something that was socially unsupported, that is, an abortion. She decided, as she put it, to "tough it out," passively opting to continue the pregnancy because abortion was, in practice, not an option.

Louisiana's ban on public funding for abortion care prevented Paige from having real access to abortion. As with the women described earlier in this chapter, Paige was affected by the ban because she was low income. Her account, though, illustrates how the opposition to abortion from her social networks increased the difficulty of overcoming the effects of the insurance ban. Had Paige been immersed in an abortion-supportive setting, raising the money for abortion may have been less difficult. Although Paige was continuing her pregnancy and now planned to parent, she was not happy to be pregnant. Just as she could not figure out how to pay for an abortion, she had no idea how she would support a baby.

Maria, a twenty-seven-year-old Hispanic woman in Louisiana, had a similar experience of her ability to choose abortion being eroded by the twin factors of structural barriers to abortion and opposition to abortion from loved ones. When Maria realized she was pregnant, she felt like it was a bad time to have a baby. Without contacting any clinics or searching online, though, Maria anticipated that the cost of an abortion would be high. She had recently relocated to Louisiana from another state, fleeing a violent relationship but having to leave behind her four children in the care of their grandmother. A psychiatrist in her home state diagnosed her with clinical depression and prescribed her medication to treat it. By the time of our interview, she had run out of pills and was waiting to see a new psychiatrist for a new prescription. She told me she felt hopeless. Unemployed, Maria had no source of funds to pay for an abortion. In some ways, this paled in comparison to her other worries, including managing her mental health, fearing violence would follow her, and anguish at being separated from her children. The man involved in this pregnancy, different from the violent man she had recently left, refused to have anything to do with the pregnancy. In their conversations, she related, he engaged in what sounds like emotional abuse. She said, "He'll tell me, you know, I'm not worth it, that he didn't want the baby and simple things like that that do hurt me."

Maria decided to seek an abortion. She hoped it would be a quick experience and not add to the many burdens she already carried. When Maria finally found a clinic and called, however, she learned that the process of obtaining an abortion in Louisiana was more involved than she expected: she would have to have two separate visits and receive state-mandated counseling. This upset her. She explained, "I thought it was just a process you say, you know, you want it done and you go in and you're going to have it done. But no, it was a process." Feeling depressed, Maria already had difficulty completing the actions needed to meet her basic needs, like grocery shopping. The prospect of multiple visits for an abortion felt overwhelming.

She had no social network resources to help her overcome feeling daunted. In fact, she experienced strong opposition to abortion from a loved one, further decreasing her ability to overcome—or even imagine overcoming—the barriers of cost and the two-visit requirement: when she told her children's grandmother that she planned to have an abortion, "she got upset with me and she told me no. She said that, if I wanted to do that, for me to let her know and she wanted to get the baby." After spending weeks unsuccessfully trying raising the money for the abortion and fielding ardent pleas for her to continue the pregnancy from her children's grandmother, the complication of having to make two visits was the straw that broke the camel's back for Maria: "I wasn't trying to wait any longer." She had no remaining emotional resources to use to navigate this obstacle. She gave up on pursuing abortion care, terrified about how she was going to raise a child by herself.

For Maria and Paige, restrictive abortion policies combined with their financial vulnerability made abortion difficult to access and therefore unchooseable. The opposition to abortion from their loved ones contributed to this outcome. As it did for Mercedes, LaToya, and Mariah, this opposition represented an absence of social network resources that they might have used to overcome structural obstacles. With a different set of social resources, these women might have had access to money to pay for an abortion and help finding a provider more promptly. That could have made a difference in their ability to choose abortion. In Paige's and Maria's experiences, opposition to abortion from others took on an ideational component as well. It represented the absence of help and, moreover, it decreased their motivation to overcome the barriers they faced. The structural barriers were real and consequential, notably affecting low-income and poor women specifically. But the barriers also gained power from the opposition to abortion from loved ones that these women encountered.

Perceived, but Illusory, Structural Obstacles

Two other Louisiana women I interviewed, like the women whose accounts have been discussed so far in this chapter, were unable to choose abortion because of structural obstacles. What was different about the obstacles they faced was that the obstacles did not concretely exist. These were not obstacles produced by policy or the organization of abortion care. They were not real obstacles at all, but these two women nonetheless perceived them as real, and, as such, they were consequential to their ability to choose abortion.

Monique, an eighteen-year-old Black woman in Louisiana, first considered abortion after her doctor mentioned it during pregnancy options counseling. As her doctor already knew, Monique had been using the hormonal contraceptive pill to prevent pregnancy and did not want to become pregnant. Her doctor estimated she was about eight weeks into her pregnancy and offered her options counseling, presenting abortion as an option for her pregnancy. In his counseling, her doctor also put a time limit on her contemplation, telling her to seek an abortion within two weeks.

That night, she told her boyfriend of three years she was pregnant. He, like her, was surprised. She did not tell him or anyone else that she was considering abortion, keeping that to herself. Then she mostly stopped thinking about the pregnancy. She told me she didn't know why she avoided thinking about the pregnancy during that time but that she "just didn't want to." For the next several weeks, Monique was in denial about her pregnancy, which meant she not only ignored the fact of her pregnancy but also refused to engage in consideration of abortion. This period exceeded the two-week clock the doctor had set for her.

Although it is unclear why the doctor presented a two-week time frame for abortion seeking, Monique believed it was because abortion was illegal in Louisiana after that point. This was not the case; Monique was still at a point in pregnancy when abortion was legal. Still, her belief that abortion was illegal and thus not available after ten weeks into pregnancy informed her consideration of abortion. She did not speak to anyone about considering abortion or seek additional information about its legality or gestational limits. Weeks later, when she was ready to confront the reality of her pregnancy, Monique thought abortion was no longer an option because "I didn't really do it within two weeks." She believed she could not legally obtain an abortion. Monique's belief that an early gestational limit in Louisiana curtailed her ability to obtain an abortion is not far-fetched. Bioethicist Michelle McGowan and colleagues (2020) argue that rapid policy changes, and the attendant media coverage, can give the impression that abortion care is unavailable when that is not the case—and this can have implications for whether individual pregnant people can obtain abortion care. At the time of our interview, Monique was nineteen weeks pregnant and still somewhat in denial about being pregnant. She had not disclosed the pregnancy to anyone other than her boyfriend.

For Shaquira, a twenty-six-year-old Black woman in Louisiana, the perceived structural obstacle consequential to her pregnancy decision making was a clinic policy related to how the fetal remains of her pregnancy would be treated. There was no such policy, but Shaquira believed there was one. That perceived but illusory obstacle made her unable to choose abortion when combined with structural barriers to abortion including the two-visit requirement as well as opposition to abortion from important others. When Shaquira first discovered she was pregnant, her reaction was immediate. She recounted, "I just didn't want to be pregnant, I didn't want to have another kid, I didn't want the responsibility, so I'm just going to go ahead and have an abortion." Shaquira had a child who was less than a year old and was surprised to have become pregnant again so soon. She did not want to have more than one child. Nor did she think it was possible to be pregnant "back to back." She said, "It's not in my genes to be so fertile." She was completely certain that abortion was the right decision for her.

Her mom, a few friends, and her partner felt differently. They opposed abortion and were vocal about it. Her partner sometimes yelled at her when they discussed abortion, and his arguments took on an aspect of emotional manipulation. Shaquira described one such conversation, saying, "At first, we were talking. The fact that we couldn't agree on it [abortion], it started to escalate into yelling, and that's when he, you know, he started saying stuff that '[you are] just so stupid.' I felt like I was stupid." Shaquira did not like what her partner was saying, and it did not persuade her that abortion was the wrong choice. She said, "I didn't feel like he knew what he was talking about. I just felt like he was just thinking about himself." Her mother, the other person she talked to about abortion repeatedly, was likewise against it. She told Shaquira several times, "You shouldn't do that."

Despite this lack of support, Shaquira made an appointment at an abortion clinic. During a break in her first appointment (of two), when she stepped outside to smoke a cigarette, she met an antiabortion protester. The protester told her, falsely, that the clinic doctor was unsafe and that the clinic would mistreat and conduct research on the fetal remains. No clinics in Louisiana donate fetal tissue to research. Shaquira, however, did not know that these asserted facts about her care were untrue and operated as though they were true. The protester's claim about conducting research on fetal remains seemed somewhat familiar, which encouraged Shaquira to believe it. In the summer of 2015, prior to Shaquira's clinic visit, antiabortion activists released covertly filmed videos of abortion providers discussing the use of fetal tissue in research, claiming that the videos showed illegal organ selling and mistreatment (Kimport and Doty 2019). Although subsequent investigations have failed to find corroborating evidence for the antiabortion activists' claims (House Committee on Oversight and Reform n.d.), the claims nonetheless entered public discourse. The inaccurate information from the protester Shaquira encountered had the practical effect of making her fearful for her safety at the clinic and upset at the idea that the fetal remains would be used in ways she did not consent to. She said that she wanted to have the remains to bury them instead, itself a practice that would be in violation of state policies on the disposition of biological material. She began to distrust the clinic personnel: "They don't tell you that they're going to give your baby to, you know, research. They don't tell you that." Believing clinic personnel would lie to her, she told me she did not ask anyone at the clinic about this practice.

While the inaccuracy of this claim is relevant to understanding Shaquira's experience, her lack of social support to navigate and manage this (false) information also mattered. Because of Louisiana's two-visit requirement and the clinic's scheduling practices,

Shaquira had a week between her first and second appointments. During that time, with important others in her life continuing to vocally oppose abortion, Shaquira had no social resources to help her make sense of her feelings about what the antiabortion protester told her. It seemed too difficult to imagine having no control over what happened to the remains of her pregnancy. Shaquira felt she could not choose abortion.

Shaquira resigned herself to continuing the pregnancy. She felt no attachment to the pregnancy, but, by five months into the pregnancy, began to feel okay about having a second child. Two months later, her circumstances changed again. Her partner was killed, leaving her a single mother to her now one-year-old son and without a co-parent for this pregnancy. She was distraught about this outcome as well as emotionally bereft about her partner's death. She said, "He was going to help me take care of the kids." She was not sure how she was going to handle everything now.

As with the real structural barriers that affected respondents' ability to choose abortion, the nonexistent policies and practices Monique and Shaquira believed to be real conditioned their ability to choose abortion. Monique believed abortion was illegal and hence unavailable to her. Shaquira believed she was required to be subject to a clinical practice she did not want. These beliefs informed their ability to choose abortion. For Shaquira, in particular, the perceived structural obstacle to abortion was powerful because it operated in a terrain already characterized by opposition to abortion by loved ones. Taken together, they made abortion something Shaquira could not choose.

After Structural Barriers

Although the women whose accounts are discussed in this chapter all stopped pursuing abortion care in response to structural barriers, not all gave up on ending their pregnancy. Three respondents from Louisiana who encountered structural barriers tried to cause an abortion outside of a medical setting. (In chapter 5, I discuss three additional cases of attempts to end pregnancy without clinical supervision, motivations for which, I argue, are distinct from those that undergird these women's actions.) Maria, described above, was despondent at the prospect of having to continue this pregnancy. Weeks after ceasing to seek abortion care, Maria attempted to end her pregnancy by consuming a bottle of over-the-counter pain medicine. She chose that medicine without much forethought: "That's what was there for me to get." It did not have the effect she desired. As she explained, "it didn't do nothing. I just got sick and started throwing up." Her attempt, nonetheless, represents the continuation of her desire to end her pregnancy, even after she stopped pursing a clinic-based abortion.

As epidemiologist Heidi Moseson and colleagues (2020) detail in their review of the literature on efforts to end a pregnancy outside of clinical supervision, there are a wide range of methods pregnant people employ, and not all are effective. Like Maria's, none of respondents' attempts was successful. Also like Maria, they tried methods of convenience, including some with no known mechanism for ending a pregnancy. I discuss their experiences less in a vein of understanding how and when such efforts can be successful and more as an illustration of the persistence of their desire to end their pregnancy as well as their agency in the face of structural barriers to clinic-based abortion. That their attempts were unsuccessful does not diminish their import. These women reacted to structural barriers with action—and with desperation. Nonetheless, the futility of their efforts—Maria's efforts made her sick but did not cause an abortion—illustrates how all-encompassing the structural barriers these women faced were.

Vanessa, a twenty-four-year-old Black woman, and her two-year-old son were homeless when she became pregnant. They had been staying on friends' couches or floors for two weeks at a time as she tried to find stable housing. The last year or so had been especially hard for Vanessa. Her fiancé, who is the father of her son, had been incarcerated. Her anxiety, anger, and bipolar disorder had been harder to manage, and sometimes she thought about suicide. She was lonely. She met a man at a friend's house who gave her comfort, and she had sex with him. She thought he used a condom but he confessed afterward that he had not. She rushed to get emergency contraception, borrowing money to pay for it from a friend because she was unable to afford it herself. Homeless, unemployed, and navigating mental health challenges, Vanessa knew she could not have a baby right now, especially not with a man who was not her fiancé. When she missed her period, she was distraught.

Vanessa quickly decided she wanted an abortion but, soon after, recognized that paying for it was beyond her financial means: "I found out I was pregnant and then I wasn't going to keep it at first. But then once [I realized] I didn't have the money for it, I was like, I have to keep it now." Vanessa first learned how expensive abortion would be when she called a clinic. When the clinic told her the cost over the phone, she demurred from scheduling an appointment, understanding that she would need time to get the money together.

Vanessa started by asking the one-night stand who had lied about using a condom for money to pay for the abortion. Rather than help her with the cost of an abortion, "he said go give the baby up for adoption." Vanessa rejected placing her baby for adoption. As for most respondents, adoption was not the alternative to abortion; parenting was. Then she called friends and family, asking for money. Anticipating opposition to abortion from others, Vanessa was vague in her explanations for why she needed the funds. Despite her concerted efforts, she was unsuccessful. She explained, "I wasn't able to get anything" from these attempts to fundraise. The people in her social networks were as financially unstable as she was, and it probably did not help that she would not specify why she needed the money.

After "trying to hustle up money" and failing, Vanessa searched online for alternatives to a clinic-based abortion. There she found recommendations that consuming large amounts of Vitamin C and amphetamine pills can cause a miscarriage. In a way, Vanessa was being resourceful: when her social networks could not help her overcome structural obstacles to a clinic-based abortion, she researched non-clinic-based abortions. This resourcefulness, though, was in response to deprivation. She had no financial resources, and her interpersonal resources—her friends and family—could not help on that front either. It is worth stating that her lack of resources was not a reflection of her worth; it was an effect of her marginalized social position. Vanessa was unemployed, with a high school education, and personally affected by racist practices of mass incarceration (Alexander 2020), which deprived her of her fiancé, and her son of his father. She tried taking Vitamin C and amphetamine pills and felt a lot of cramping, but "it didn't do nothing." Increasingly despondent, Vanessa described "feeling like punching my stomach sometimes." Her existing mental health difficulties grew worse.

As Vanessa completed the first trimester of her pregnancy, she was resigned to the fact that she could not choose abortion. She could not afford a clinic-based abortion, and her attempts at ending the pregnancy on her own had failed. About fifteen weeks into her pregnancy, she confessed to her fiancé that she was pregnant. He was angry. Vanessa feared he might end their relationship but accepted this possibility. By the time of our interview, four weeks after she told her fiancé, he had softened and told Vanessa that he was open to being a father to this child. Vanessa, however, did not feel relieved. She was still homeless, struggling to feed herself and her son, and only saw things getting harder once this baby was born.

Kara, a twenty-two-year-old Black woman in Louisiana, also attempted—and failed—to end her pregnancy after structural obstacles to abortion made it impossible for her to choose a clinic-based abortion. In her case, the power of these structural obstacles was magnified by opposition to abortion from loved ones. Kara knew upon discovering her pregnancy that she did not want to continue it and, from a friend's experience of abortion, knew that it would be expensive. Overt opposition to abortion from her boyfriend and her mother, accompanied by softer opposition from her older niece, to whom she was very close, informed Kara's abortion consideration. Although her roommate was supportive and even encouraging of her consideration of abortion, Kara centrally sought the support of her boyfriend and immediate family. Facing only their clear hostility to abortion, Kara felt sad and was unsure how to cope with her pregnancy. She hoped that it would "go away."

She was also wary of the costs—both financial and reputational—of going to a clinic for an abortion. Currently a student, Kara was certain she could not afford a clinic-based abortion and was uncertain she could handle what visiting an abortion clinic would mean to her and others who found out. She said, "I really didn't want to go to a clinic, and I knew it would be a lot of money that goes into that." Still, she did not want to be pregnant.

With a clinic-based abortion unavailable to her, Kara turned to the Internet for solutions, searching for non-clinic-based ways to end a pregnancy. She explained, "I looked it up online. It was really like home remedies or natural ways." Among the ways to cause an abortion Kara found online "were a few suggestions that like taking a really, really hot bath or a really, really hot shower, or I think it was one that said drink a lot of—I don't know. They really didn't make sense after a while." Even so, Kara "did try the shower thing a couple of times."

In addition, in part hoping it would make the pregnancy go away and in part just trying to cope, Kara drank alcohol, believing that since it is discouraged for pregnant people, it might cause a miscarriage: "I tried having a drink every now and again, hoping that it would go away." She described drinking three or so drinks twice a week for the first several weeks after she discovered her pregnancy. The only effect it had was to make her sick. Taking hot showers was also unsuccessful. As time passed, Kara came to recognize that she could not be successful ending the pregnancy on her own. By ten weeks gestation, she stopped drinking alcohol and engaging in other efforts to cause a miscarriage.

In effect, Maria, Vanessa, and Kara, all in Louisiana, were trying to work around the structural barriers to abortion they encountered. They attempted to end their pregnancies on their own after facing, and perhaps in response to, substantial structural barriers to abortion. Certainly, they represented the minority of women I interviewed, but these cases illustrate how respondents' implicit recognition of how structural barriers made clinic-based abortion unchooseable was not equivalent to acquiescence to continuing their pregnancies. These attempts show women's agency as well as how difficult structural barriers can be to surmount.

Conclusion

In their accounts of considering but not obtaining an abortion, many of the respondents described a structural barrier that was consequential to their decision making. This sounds like a familiar story. As the introductory chapter detailed, the effect of abortion-restrictive policies in preventing pregnant people from obtaining a wanted abortion is well evidenced. Here, I offer additional support for these findings and extend that literature by illustrating that—and how—structures can serve as barriers for pregnant people who do not ever contact an abortion provider. The effect of structural barriers on people's ability to obtain an abortion is likely even more extensive than the literature to date has found. Structures related to restrictive policies and the organization of abortion care affected the ability of these pregnant women to choose abortion before they made it to a clinic. Although respondents in both Louisiana and Maryland faced structural barriers to abortion, women in Louisiana were more likely to not obtain an abortion after considering one because of a policy-related reason (S. Roberts, Kimport, et al. 2019). As I show in this chapter, however, this finding does not mean that Maryland women faced no structural barriers to abortion.

What these structures did was make choosing abortion impossible for these respondents. Without money or insurance coverage to pay for abortion, abortion was unchooseable. Without a provider, without adequate time off to meet the two-visit requirement (which only applied to the Louisiana respondents), or without transportation to a provider, abortion was unchooseable. Without social support to navigate these obstacles, abortion was unchooseable.

These structural barriers did not, it bears specifying, make respondents want to have a baby. Nor did they contribute to ensuring that these women could parent in safe and sustainable communities, a central principle of reproductive justice (Ross et al. 2017). Several of the women whose accounts are discussed in this chapter experienced violence from partners and parents. Several reported living in unsafe communities, and a few were homeless. Structural barriers made abortion unchooseable but failed to provide the resources to make parenting in a safe community possible.

I have also drilled into the sources of the "withouts" so many respondents faced. They were without money, transportation, and flexible work schedules because they were low income and poor. And because they were low income and poor and had to rely on support from others to surmount existing obstacles, opposition to abortion from loved ones was acutely consequential. It was their poverty, then, that was a central contributor to their inability to choose abortion. That poverty for the Black respondents was connected to historical and contemporary racist policy that perpetuates income and wealth inequality by race. The fact that abortion was unchooseable for them is therefore tied to their social location as Black women who are financially struggling. The women described in this chapter lacked access to the resources, both material and interpersonal, that could enable them to overcome structural obstacles to abortion; abortion was unchooseable. And, for this reason, despite their desire not to, they were continuing their pregnancies.

3

Privileging the Fetus

While the experiences of women like Jayla, who encountered both financial and gestational barriers to abortion, and Tyler, who could not negotiate adequate time off from work to complete Louisiana's two-visit requirement during her first trimester, have been studied and measured in the research literature, considerably less attention has been paid to how the ability to choose abortion can be constrained by nonstructural obstacles as well. This is what happened to respondents like Courtney. Courtney, a twenty-one-year-old Black woman in Louisiana, never presented for abortion care and did not know about the restrictions on abortion in Louisiana. It is likely that some of those restrictions would have proved to be a hardship for her: Courtney relied on public insurance, so the ban on public insurance coverage of abortion would have affected her, and she had inflexible work hours, making the two-visit requirement also a potential obstacle. But Courtney's ability to choose abortion was constrained before these structural obstacles could even come up.

Courtney had not envisioned herself ever becoming a parent. That life plan was complicated when she learned she was pregnant, and she thought abortion could be the right choice for her. Each person she talked to about her pregnancy and desire for abortion, however, responded by negating her desire with an assertion that abortion is killing. For example, when Courtney told her boyfriend she was pregnant, she related, "he was like 'oh my god. Don't kill it.' Because he, I guess, he felt like I would get an abortion." Her boyfriend was not alone in ardently discouraging abortion by defining it as killing. When Courtney told her mother she was considering abortion, "she was like no. She was just not with it at all. She was just like, 'No, you're not doing that.'" Courtney's sister said the same. As Courtney summed it up, "Everybody basically was just like 'no.'" As she explained, "My family, we really don't believe in abortions or killing babies at all." Courtney's articulation of the meaning of abortion as killing was tethered to a sense of her identity and what her family stands for. Nodding to an implied and felt as real family belief, Courtney explained that these interactions with loved ones reminded her of this foundational belief that abortion represents killing and compelled her to apply it to her current pregnancy decision making.

At the time of our interview, when she was six months pregnant, Courtney described how her thinking about abortion changed over time. She explained, "As time progressed, I didn't think that [abortion] was the right decision for me. And I'm a good person and I feel like I can deal with having a child and taking and raising my child." She elaborated about abortion: "I feel like you're killing it. I feel like you're killing it even when you find out that you're pregnant. Because it's a life that you created." Certainly, not everyone who considers abortion proceeds to abortion. In Courtney's case, though, the shift in her thinking was prompted by a change in what abortion meant to her. As important people in her life insisted over and over again that abortion was killing, it became harder to choose, especially since, as Courtney insisted, "I'm a good person." When the available social meaning for abortion positions it as morally wrong—not what a good person would choose—choosing abortion means challenging one's sense of self. Courtney held to her identity as a good person and, in so doing, decided she could not choose abortion.

At play in Courtney's account are cultural narratives about the meaning of abortion. Cultural narratives convey broad social meanings and can define the terrain within which abortion decision making takes place. In practice, narratives are rooted in the cultural imagination: they represent the contours of how people in particular spaces and communities make sense of the world. As Courtney's experience illustrates, respondents engaged with narratives about abortion in their pregnancy decision making. It was into these extant meanings that respondents waded as they contemplated abortion and their pregnancy. Many of those narratives oriented the meaning of abortion around ideas about the fetus and potential life. In this chapter, I focus on those cultural narratives; in the following chapter, I examine narratives that constructed meanings of abortion related to the person seeking an abortion.

For each set of narratives—those about the fetus and those about the pregnant person—I trace its operation in respondents' lives and pregnancy decision making, highlighting how these narratives motivated some respondents to (in)action. The inability to imagine how one could choose abortion meant, for many respondents, that abortion was unchooseable. In practice, these cultural narratives operated not just as ways of understanding abortion but as barriers to choosing abortion. And, in turn, when abortion was unchooseable, respondents also lacked the opportunity to choose under what circumstances they wanted to have a baby. Additionally, I trace the rhetorical construction and origins of these cultural narratives. Although the two sets of narratives differed in their general content, both have their origins in antiabortion ideology and social movements, pointing to an extralegal mechanism through which political and social contention over abortion has infiltrated individual women's pregnancy decision making.

Abortion as Killing

A key feature of Courtney's understanding of the meaning of abortion was a cultural narrative that defined abortion as killing. This idea was common across the interviews with women from both Louisiana and Maryland. As an example, Mikela, a twenty-seven-year-old Black woman in Louisiana, became pregnant from a casual relationship with a friend. When she discovered her pregnancy, she did not want to continue it. In part, this stemmed from her expectations that the man involved would not be an engaged parent. She had a very close relationship with her father, and she wanted the same for her children. This man was unlikely to fulfill that role. In fact, they had already stopped seeing each other before Mikela learned she was pregnant. This made her unhappy about her pregnancy. She explained, "I didn't want my baby to grow up without a father." Mikela also had concerns about her ability to carry a healthy pregnancy. For the past few years, she had been grappling with chronic nausea that her doctors had been unable to explain or treat. The nausea was debilitating. Mikela reported that "sometimes, I wake up and just cry because I feel so bad." To give context to her use of "sometimes," I asked how often it gets that bad, and she related, "I mean five times a day it'll get bad." On a recent occasion when she went to the emergency room because she could not stop vomiting, they gave her a pregnancy test. Getting a positive result was shocking for Mikela. She said, "I started shaking. I started getting weak. It was unexpected. And I got scared because I was telling him [the doctor] I don't eat on my own. I don't know how it's going to work. I don't want [the baby] to come out not grown and stuff." Her doctor referred her to prenatal care.

Mikela mulled over abortion but had doubts that she could choose it. She accepted the idea of her pregnancy as already a child and therefore understood abortion to mean a harm against her own child. She also invoked the idea of the potential life she carried as innocent, saying of her pregnancy, "My child don't have nothing to do with this. It didn't ask to be here. So, it's not right to get rid of it [have an abortion]. That's not right. And, that'll be heavy on my heart." Without talking to anyone about her consideration of abortion, operating in discursive terrain dominated by belief that abortion was harming her child, Mikela determined that abortion was unchooseable for her pregnancy.

Mikela's reasons for considering abortion, however, remained: her nausea continued unabated and unexplained, and her expectations about the man involved came true. When she told him about the pregnancy, she said, it "scared him off." She had not spoken with him in the month since telling him about the pregnancy and believed he had moved out of state. At the time of our interview, she felt no excitement for her pregnancy. She explained, "I can't really get excited . . . because my child's going to grow up without a dad, and I don't want that." Not only was abortion unchooseable for Mikela, she was also unable to choose the circumstances under which she wanted to parent.

Mikela's experience of finding it impossible to fully consider choosing abortion under a rubric of the fetus as a person was not unique. With a new baby at home and not expecting to be pregnant, Martina, a twenty-five-year-old Black woman in Maryland, got confirmation of her pregnancy from her doctor when she was thirteen weeks pregnant. Considering her fetus a person at that gestational stage, she explained that abortion was now unacceptable: "As far as abortion because, you know, who wants to get an abortion when they're [three], four months pregnant, five months pregnant? You know what I mean? You still think of it as a baby. It's a lot harder to go ahead with that decision [than] when you're so much earlier. It's a whole baby. You know what I mean?" Understanding her fetus to be equivalent to a person, Martina found abortion unchooseable. It felt intuitively wrong. Martina's sense of this belief as a collectively accepted standard, as evidenced in her question "You know what I mean?," points to the way this narrative about what abortion means seemed like common sense. As such, Martina felt like abortion was broadly unchooseable.

THE CONTOURS OF THE ABORTION AS KILLING NARRATIVE

In Martina's, Mikela's, and Courtney's accounts, the idea that abortion is killing featured heavily. This idea was nearly ubiquitous among the interviewees. Morgan, a twenty-seven-year-old Black woman in Maryland, was concise, stating simply, "I just look at abortion as murder." Deirdre, a thirty-year-old Black woman in Maryland, asserted that, with abortion, "the reality [is] that you're getting rid of a life. That's something big." The construction of abortion as killing was premised on the idea of the fetus as a person, what is termed "fetal personhood" in the literature. Selena, a twenty-five-year-old Black woman in Maryland, explained that "it's just not right to kill something. I feel like it's a person, whether it's a fetus or whatever you want to call it, it's just a person." Under a logic of the fetus as a person, abortion was constructed as inherently morally wrong. ·

There was some variation in when respondents considered fetal personhood established. For Noreen, a thirty-eight-year-old Black woman in Louisiana, personhood began when there were fetal heart tones, which typically start around six weeks into pregnancy: "There was a heartbeat [sic] with these babies at six to seven weeks. I feel like that's a life. It's something that is formed. Something is actually living." Samantha, a thirty-eight-year-old white woman in Maryland, assigned fetal personhood after ten weeks gestation. As she summed up, at ten weeks, to her "it was a whole baby in there and not just a blob." Across the interviews, although they varied in the point in pregnancy at which fetal personhood emerged, most respondents constructed fetal personhood as objectively identifiable and absolute. It existed at and after a certain point.

This idea of an embryo or fetus as the equivalent of an independently living person is not distinctive of these respondents. Scholars have documented the pervasive conceptualization of fetal personhood among pregnant people and others around them (Layne 2003; L. Morgan and Michaels 1999). Research has also demonstrated that this belief in fetal personhood is constructed, not innate. Attribution of personhood to the fetus as well as to young infants has varied by historical and cultural context (Dubow 2010; L. Morgan 2009), but has found ready purchase in the contemporary moment. Scholars have attributed this rise in belief in fetal personhood to the advent and subsequent ubiquity of ultrasound images of the fetus (Dubow 2010; Taylor 1992, 2008). Such disembodied images, often presented without cues to scale, have been used to emphasize the similarities between a fetus and a newborn baby in a range of cultural settings including popular culture and advertising (Layne 2000). In the setting of the obstetrical ultrasound, these images are typically accompanied by language socializing pregnant people and their partners into the social role of parent and naming the fetus as their "baby" (Mitchell and

Georges 1998). Other scholars have argued that medical advances like fetal surgery (Casper 1998), prenatal antismoking campaigns (Oaks 2001), and prenatal care itself (C. Williams, Alderson, and Farsides 2001) have informed attribution of fetal personhood. Collectively, these biomedical interventions have contributed to the ability to define the fetus as a person. This framing, Lavin (2001) argues, has been especially resonant in the United States because of its culture of privileging of the individual.

WHEN KILLING IS ALLOWABLE

There was some nuance in respondents' application of this cultural narrative of abortion as killing. Several women explained that they considered abortion killing but would still support abortion under certain circumstances. Selena, who described abortion as killing and not right, also asserted that abortion would be acceptable if the person seeking one "had a legitimate reason. . . . It would have to either have a medical reason or they would have to have a real reason why they want the abortion." When I asked her what she meant by "real reason," she elaborated: "If they couldn't afford another baby, I guess it would be a real reason in a way. Because, they don't want the baby to be poor. They don't want to have the baby, and the baby don't have the right stuff to take care of them, so I guess that would be a real reason. But, they can't just come in there and say they just don't want it or that it was a mistake." Selena generated an expansive list of acceptable reasons, but her insistence on there being acceptable and unacceptable reasons for abortion was rooted in narratives privileging potential life. Her default construction of abortion was as killing, but she stated that it could be morally acceptable when it was sought for certain reasons.

Other respondents echoed this idea that particular reasons for abortion would weigh against their overall disapproval of abortion on fetal grounds. Aliyah, an eighteen-year-old Black woman in Maryland whose account is detailed later in this chapter, believed that abortion was killing and against God's will but explained that she would support a friend seeking an abortion if—and only if—her friend could offer a "good reason," which, she explained, included, "she is living on the street or something like that." Others who considered abortion killing were far more narrow in their allowances of when abortion could be morally acceptable, mostly restricting their acceptance to pregnancies that resulted from rape. This is consistent with public opinion trends wherein people report greater support for abortion in instances of rape than for other reasons (Jozkowski, Crawford, and Hunt 2018; Smith and Son 2013). Tara, a twenty-one-year-old Black woman in Maryland, for instance, was emphatic that she was okay with abortion only in some narrowly defined cases, and went so far as to be prescriptive in those cases. Specifically, she said, "the only thing I think people that should have abortions is people that have problems and rape or something bad happened to them."

In these ways, although some respondents understood the cultural narrative of abortion as killing in a nuanced way, they still preserved the formulation that abortion is killing. Their willingness to offer exceptions defined by the reason the pregnant person sought the abortion did not disrupt the narrative's construction of abortion as killing. Rather, it carved out exceptions for when killing was allowable—and none of the respondents whose pregnancy decision making was affected by the abortion as killing narrative saw themselves in those exceptions.

THE ROLE OF THE ANTIABORTION MOVEMENT

This construction of the fetus as a person and of abortion as killing owes to the concerted efforts of antiabortion activists. Although the term "antiabortion activist" often conjures an image of someone engaged in direct action, such as a street protest at a clinic, the antiabortion movement has also engaged in extensive efforts to remake policy and cultural ideas about abortion (Mason 2002). Soon after the 1973 *Roe v. Wade* decision, antiabortion advocates sought a constitutional amendment defining fetuses as persons and abortion as murder (Hull and Hoffer 2010; Petchesky 1984), a hope that never materialized. In the years since, the antiabortion movement has sought to frame the fetus as a baby in public discourse (Doan 2007; Mason 2002; Ziegler 2015) and to strategically construct abortion as murder (Schoen 2015). Sociologist Rosalind Petchesky (1984, 1987) characterizes this movement strategy as an effort to move attention away from the voices and experiences of women, effectively silencing them as subjects in the political debate on abortion (see also Reagan 1997).

Scholars have traced this effort on several fronts. Antiabortion activists have deployed fetal imagery in mass culture, from video to sonogram images, to assert fetal personhood and construct abortion as murder in a conscious effort to win over the public (Petchesky 1987; Taylor 1992). Likewise, they have forwarded legislation grounded in this framework, including laws not ostensibly related to abortion, such as fetal homicide and fetal pain laws (Halva-Neubauer and Zeigler 2010), and laws focused on abortion, such as the 2003 federal "Partial Birth Abortion Ban" (Ludlow 2008) and mandatory pre-abortion ultrasound viewing laws (Andaya and Mishtal 2017). In this legislation, the debates surrounding its passage, and the judicial decisions on its constitutionality, the record reflects language asserting and naturalizing innate fetal personhood, using, for example, the word "child" instead of "fetus" (Andaya and Mishtal 2017; Halva-Neubauer and Zeigler 2010; Ludlow 2008).

As this framing has entered public discourse, the cultural narrative of abortion as killing has gained traction and, as Petchesky (1984, 1987) anticipated, the voices of people who have abortions have been erased. Public health scientist Katie Woodruff (2019), for instance, shows that media coverage of abortion in the United States commonly personifies the fetus. Woodruff's analysis also illustrates a parallel occurrence: the decentering of the circumstances of people who seek abortions. Media coverage is more likely to personify the fetus than to report on abortion experiences from actual women. In other words, the framing of the fetus as inherently a person has received greater public attention than the embodied experiences of pregnant people and their social relationships to the pregnancy. In these ways, the increasing dominance of a frame of inherent fetal personhood has been coupled with the erasure of the circumstances and experiences of pregnant people

at the level of public discourse. Rhetorically, this serves to frag-
ment the fetus from the pregnant person, making it possible for
the fetus to retain personhood status and deflecting attention from
the pregnant person's authority to make decisions about the
pregnancy.

God's Infallibility and Intentionality

Respondents invoked another narrative of abortion that focused
on the fetus, one that opposed abortion based on belief in their
god's infallibility and intentionality. Kendra, a thirty-three-year-
old Black woman in Maryland, was raising seven children. Less
than a year before our interview, Kendra had been laid off from a
secure job and could no longer afford her rent. Six months before
our interview, she and her children moved into a homeless shelter.
Kendra had been celibate for three years when she decided to have
sex with a friend one weekend. The condom broke. First thing the
next morning, Kendra went to the hospital for emergency contraception, only to be told it was available in the emergency room
solely for rape victims. The local clinic that would provide it for
free was not open during the weekend. When she called them the
following Monday, they "would not give me an appointment until
that Friday," by which time Kendra knew emergency contraception would not be effective: "You got to take it within the first three
days." She decided to chance it, worrying about the possibility of
pregnancy but rationalizing that her chances were low. When her
period did not come a few weeks later, she realized she was
pregnant.

Years prior, soon after her third child was born, Kendra had
two abortions. Each time, she felt certain abortion was the right
decision and did not have moral concerns about it. In the time
since, however, her discussions with her mother and oldest brother
changed her thinking. She said, "I felt like I realized that abortions are bad. Prior to that, I didn't really know that abortion was
bad." Asked what prompted this change, she elaborated, "I got
reading and seeking God more, that's all. And it said in the Bible

'He knew me before I was in my mother's womb.'" Kendra interpreted this as evidence of God-given personhood before conception, and that abortion was therefore a sin against God. She promised herself she would not have another abortion.

Still, Kendra felt conflicted about her current pregnancy: "I was just mad because I was like, good grief, look at this. I'm like, who gets pregnant and homeless?" Despite her prior promise, she could not figure out how she would support eight children, especially without stable housing. Referencing her understanding that her religion prohibited abortion, she said, "I was trying to talk to God and see if I could get an abortion even though, you know, I don't believe in abortion." One day when she was praying, she remembered the smell of the room after her abortions. She said this reminded her of her commitment to God not to have another: "It was just a memory and [reminded me] that I need to take control over my feelings instead of allowing my feelings to control me."

The first month after she discovered her pregnancy, Kendra thought often about abortion but, each time, stopped herself from fully considering it. She said, "I wouldn't really dwell on it because, I think, in my mind I'm like, you know you ain't going to get no abortion. What about your promise and your commitment?" Although Kendra kept coming back to the idea of abortion, her belief that her god was hostile to abortion prevented her from choosing it. For Kendra, choosing abortion meant going against her religious beliefs and doing something that was inconsistent with her sense of herself as a moral person. Choosing abortion required overcoming the obstacles of imagination that the cultural narrative of abortion as against God's will had erected. Understandably, Kendra could not do this. For Kendra, abortion was unchooseable.

Other respondents, too, believed in a divine intention behind their pregnancy. Rashida, a thirty-one-year-old Black woman in Maryland, had recently moved and was proud that her new home meant each of her three sons got his own room. She was also struggling with debt, chronic neck pain, an autoimmune disorder, feelings of depression and isolation, and, recently, panic attacks and fainting. After passing out for unknown reasons, Rashida left her most recent job; she feared passing out again and what it would mean for her safety. When she discovered she was pregnant, Rashida felt scared. She explained: "This time it was kind of scary. [I] didn't know what to do. I had mixed feelings. I wanted the baby, didn't want the baby, [would] think I wasn't ready for the baby. It's all part of mixed feelings. I just moved and I was like, I don't know. I feel like all kids [should] have their own room. I'm not rich. I'm just going through so much." On top of those feelings and pressures, Rashida was certain that continuing her pregnancy would impede her ability to get a job: "Nobody going to hire me when I'm pregnant." Centering her own health and her existing children's needs, Rashida "felt like it [abortion] was the right decision because like as far as financially . . . at least I can take care of them [my children]. I can provide for them."

Yet these assessments were only part of her evaluation of her situation. She also thought of pregnancy as natural and sanctioned by a higher power. She believed that God would not make her pregnant unless he wanted her to continue the pregnancy. As she explained: "I'm not religio[us], but I do believe in God. I just believe in one person. I feel like everybody got one person. They just choose to call him different names and that's fine. I feel like he wouldn't have kept giving me the babies if he didn't want me to have the babies. That's just how I felt." In this same vein, Rashida referenced her recent history of two abortions as further evidence that God wanted her to have another baby. She said, "Okay, we getting two abortions and then I still end up pregnant? It was like, what was the reason that you got two abortions and you still end up [pregnant] again?" Rashida adopted a fatalistic logic. Even as she articulated health and family reasons why she should not continue her pregnancy, her cultural understanding of her pregnancy was that it was intended by God. Under this belief system, Rashida understood abortion as denying God's will that she have another child. For her, this understanding made abortion unchooseable.

Both Kendra and Rashida thought about abortion in a context of their Christian god's infallibility and intentionality. (All of the respondents who considered themselves religious adhered to a form of Christianity; see the Methodological Appendix.) As Mariah, from chapter 2, stated, God was infallible: "I believe that God made no mistakes." He was, further, intentional. Mercedes, also from chapter 2, explained, "I believe that God does things in your life for a reason, even if it's good or bad. You've just got to know how to work through them obstacles." As Taylor, a twenty-six-year-old Black woman in Louisiana, succinctly said, "Everything happens for a reason." Similarly, Tandra, a thirty-four-year-old Black woman in Louisiana, said, "If [something] happens, it's for a reason and I know God is not going to put something on me that I can't bear."

It was not just respondents themselves who invoked this narrative of divine determination. Loved ones in respondents' lives cited these beliefs as well. For example, when Shaunice, a twenty-one-year-old Black woman in Louisiana, told her sister about her pregnancy, her sister assured her, "God wouldn't give you more than you can handle." LaToya, from chapter 2, related that she had heard this sentiment often: "My family always said that he [God] wouldn't put anything on you that you couldn't handle or something like that." This narrative of divine infallibility and intentionality, in other words, was a pervasive way in which respondents made sense of their world. These women understood events in their lives as purposeful, as directed by God, even if they did not understand the purpose in the moment.

In practice, respondents did not apply a narrative of divine intentionality and infallibility to every experience in their lives. Sometimes, they reasoned, things just happen. But they and others consistently applied this narrative of intentionality to make sense of their pregnancies. Sequitta, a thirty-eight-year-old Black woman in Maryland, reported of her grandmother that she "is telling me that that [my pregnancy] is God's child. God put the baby for a reason." Noreen, introduced above, related the response from an acquaintance when she told her of this pregnancy: "She said, 'Take it as a blessing because things happen for a reason.'" Noreen struggled with this framework, noting, "I'm still trying to figure this reason out," but also trusted God, expecting to recognize the reason for her pregnancy in time.

Key to this narrative was a second construction of God's will: that God wanted the respondent to continue the pregnancy and have a baby. The narrative did not, in other words, only assert intentionality behind the pregnancy. It also constructed abortion as negating God's intention. Erasing the possibility of abortion as a pregnancy outcome, Aliyah, whose experience is described in detail below, said, "If he did not want me to have this child, then he would, you know, I would maybe have a miscarriage or I mean I would have not even got pregnant. So, it's all for a reason."

It is interesting to note that these women did not suggest that they lacked the ability to end their pregnancies. Despite religious arguments about the Christian god being the only one with agency to make determinations over life and death, these women stipulated that they were theoretically able to choose abortion and, in a logic of abortion as killing, cause death. What they grappled with was whether they could make this choice, given their understanding of the meaning of abortion. This narrative constructed abortion as against God's will, compelling an understanding of abortion as something they should not choose and therefore could not choose. Like the abortion as killing narrative, the infallible God narrative, in effect, constructed abortion as unchooseable.

THE ROLE OF THE ANTIABORTION MOVEMENT

While respondents understood a prohibition on abortion to be definitional of their religious faith, not all religions are opposed to abortion. Indeed, not even all Christian denominations are opposed to abortion (Hoffmann and Johnson 2005). Nor have the denominations now opposed to abortion always been vocally so (Hoffmann and Johnson 2005; Reagan 1997). In the 1960s, as state legislatures debated abortion decriminalization and legalization, the Catholic Church was the only institution to mount a campaign in opposition (Haugeberg 2017). This time period also marked the Church's first coordinated messaging on abortion, with Catholic bishops formulating antiabortion messaging that was then disseminated by parish priests (D. Williams 2015a). The Catholic Church had not previously coordinated its teachings in opposition to abortion, suggesting that abortion had not previously been a central focus.

It was not until the 1970s that evangelicals and some mainline Protestant denominations began to actively identify with the antiabortion movement and frame abortion as against religious tenets. Prior to this point, historian David K. Williams (2015b) argues, mainline Protestants and evangelicals were largely uninvolved in antiabortion activism because they did not uniformly consider abortion—or all abortions—to be wrong (see also Holland 2020). Indeed, at several of their conventions in the 1970s, the Southern Baptists passed resolutions in support of abortion in some circumstances (Ammerman 1990). As sociologist Nancy Ammerman (1990) charts, by 1980, that had shifted. Evangelical leaders increasingly adopted a rigid antiabortion position.

Historian Jennifer Holland (2020) demonstrates that this shift was not exclusively top-down and, further, was connected to racist ideology. Members of religious congregations pushed their clergy leaders to make public proclamations against abortion and engage their congregations in prolife actions, particularly in Catholic, Mormon, and evangelical congregations. Holland ties this effort and its effect of associating Christianity with opposition to abortion to a politics of whiteness. She traces how white social conservatives' desire to claim moral authority in the wake of the legacy of slavery and ongoing racism latched onto abortion, enabling white people to claim to be "modern-day 'abolitionists'" by opposing abortion, without having to revisit extant racist policies and practices that privilege whiteness. In so doing, these lay activists politicized religious spaces and speech, rendering opposition to abortion central to many Christian religious identities and, as clergy leaders adopted these efforts, denominations. The understanding of abortion as inherently opposed by Christian religious teachings is neither absolute nor historically true. This cultural narrative is a product of specific political efforts, grounded in a white socially conservative identity.

Race, Class, and the Impacts of Constructing Abortion as Morally Wrong

Although many respondents and others in their lives drew on the infallible God narrative to construct becoming pregnant as something beyond their control, becoming pregnant when you do not expect to be is not a randomly distributed experience. It is patterned. Black women at any income level are more likely than white women to become pregnant when they did not plan to be, and low-income Black women, in particular, are most likely to experience an unintended pregnancy (Dehlendorf et al. 2010; Finer and Zolna 2016).

Physician-researcher Christine Dehlendorf and colleagues (2010) identify three factors that contribute to this outcome. At the individual level, they note differences in women's preferences and behaviors, including differences in contraceptive method preferences, level of medical mistrust, and knowledge about reproductive health and contraception. Some of these differences, such as a higher level of medical mistrust among Black women, are rooted in the racist history of reproductive medicine's experimentation on the bodies of women of color and experiences of medical racism (see chapter 1). At the level of interaction, Dehlendorf and colleagues identify provider-related factors, such as implicit bias, that interfere with meeting patient needs. Medical providers treat family planning patients differently based on race and income (Stevens 2015) and may pressure low-income women and women of color to use particular methods that may or may not meet their preferences (Downing, LaVeist, and Bullock 2007; Mann 2013; Thorburn and Bogart 2005). Finally, the authors identify healthcare system factors, such as differences in access to insurance and coverage of contraception. Both historically and in the contemporary moment, Black people have higher rates of being uninsured compared to white people (Artiga, Orgera, and Damico 2020), which can impact their ability to secure contraception that meets their needs (Ebrahim et al. 2009). Each of these contributors to the disproportionate rate of unintended pregnancy among low-income Black women itself is an effect of and builds on structural inequalities of race and class. Because of race and class inequality, low-income Black women are more likely than other groups to become pregnant when they do not want to be.

To the extent that consideration of abortion is more common in response to a pregnancy that was not expected, it is then low-income Black women who are most likely to be in a position where they consider abortion. It is their voices, their personal evaluations, and their autonomy that the fetus-focused cultural narratives of abortion supersede and devalue in pregnancy decision making. Moreover, in the process, the operation of structural inequalities, as well as discrimination by providers and the healthcare system, is erased and its effects naturalized. The question of why respondents were pregnant when they did not want to be—and the role of race and class inequality in producing this outcome—is displaced. These antiabortion cultural constructions of abortion direct attention away from the pregnant person's circumstances and the social structures that produced those circumstances. As the following accounts illustrate, in so doing, they can make abortion unchooseable.

Narratives of the Fetus and Potential Life in Action

Aliyah and Valencia each initially decided they wanted an abortion for their unexpected pregnancy. After subsequent exposure to fetus-focused antiabortion cultural narratives, both of abortion as killing and of abortion as against God's will, however, neither felt able to choose abortion under the ideational constraints of these narratives. Even as both expected to continue their pregnancies, the narratives that made abortion unchooseable did not compel feelings of attachment.

Aliyah, introduced above, began her pregnancy decision making by attending to her thoughts on the pregnancy and becoming a parent. At that point, she did not want to be pregnant. She was in her final year of high school and felt unprepared to have a baby, especially because she was estranged from her mother. She could not imagine becoming a mother when she felt so negatively about her own mother. Recounting her thinking at that time, she said, "That's the first thing that came to mind: I want an abortion because I did not want to deal with those personal issues at home and then also because I just thought it wasn't a good time." Aliyah and her boyfriend agreed abortion was the right choice. She called a clinic and scheduled an appointment, feeling, she said, "a lot" of certainty that abortion was the right decision for her. Then she spoke with some family members who insisted on a different meaning for abortion, one that privileged the fetus and potential life.

Aliyah told her sister, cousin, and aunt of her plan to obtain an abortion. While her sister's response was generally neutral, both her aunt and her cousin voiced strong opposition to abortion that invoked their religion and defined abortion as killing. Aliyah described her conversation with her aunt: "I first talked to my aunt [about abortion] because my aunt is like my mother, a mother to me, and she was telling me, well, because part of my religion, we aren't really supposed to kill babies." In citing their Christian faith, Aliyah's aunt positioned Aliyah's consideration of abortion as opposed to their religiously informed understanding of abortion as killing a baby. Aliyah's cousin concurred.

Aliyah found her relatives' framing persuasive. As described above, Aliyah believed that everything, including—and perhaps specifically—her pregnancy, happens for a reason, so her relatives' claims resonated with her. She shifted her thinking about her pregnancy, no longer privileging what she wanted or what she felt was best for her and instead evaluating those reasons against a narrative of abortion as killing. She could not imagine killing someone, especially not for the reasons she had been considering abortion. Thinking about what her aunt and cousin had said made her realize, she explained, that "I should not kill an innocent baby because of myself or maybe because of issues with my mother." She was no longer trying to decide whether she could parent under her current circumstances. Instead, her evaluation was about whether she should—and, in turn, could—choose abortion, under a definition of abortion as killing and against her god's will.

These frameworks of abortion as morally wrong undermined Aliyah's ability to assert the validity of her consideration of abortion. When her aunt challenged her reasons for abortion, Aliyah capitulated: "She was telling me I can't [have an abortion] and I really didn't have a good reason. I really didn't." Aliyah did not have a reason to continue the pregnancy either. But that was not the calculus her loved ones presented to her. Aliyah was deciding whether she could choose abortion. And she decided, given the meanings of abortion advanced by the cultural narratives of abortion as killing and as against God's will, that she could not. She called the abortion clinic and canceled her appointment.

In the time since Aliyah decided she could not choose abortion, her relationship with her mother had further deteriorated, and she had moved in with her aunt. Her aunt promised to help take care of the baby when it was born, and Aliyah had plans to get a job. Overall, she said, "I'm happy, especially right now with just baby planning," but she had chosen not to disclose her pregnancy to anyone else. She said she planned to eventually but anticipated they would not be supportive, saying, "I just, right now, don't really feel like dealing with that." Her boyfriend had accepted that she was continuing the pregnancy. He said he would take a parenting class, but he was vague about when. Aliyah was unsure what resources she would need to support a baby, but hopeful that she could find them and that she and her boyfriend would be able to do "what we originally planned on way before the baby came," including college and trade school. What it would mean to become a parent remained abstract for Aliyah. And although she had warmed to the idea of becoming a parent, she did not feel especially connected to her pregnancy.

Like Aliyah, Valencia, a thirty-five-year-old Black and Mexican woman in Maryland, described a shift in her pregnancy decision making as she was exposed to antiabortion cultural narratives. When Valencia discovered her pregnancy, she felt like it was a difficult time to bring a child into the family. She was a full-time caregiver for her four children as well as the primary caregiver for her grandparents. Her husband was the only one working in their household of ten, encompassing her nuclear family, her sister and brother-in-law, and her grandparents. As Valencia related, "It can be overwhelming with a husband that works and four kids and yelling and screaming. And then, I deal with my elderly grandparents and taking care of them." Her first feeling about the pregnancy was that she should seek an abortion. She said, "I just thought having another one [child] wouldn't be a good time right now." It would not be her first abortion. She had four prior abortions, each under different circumstances.

When she told her husband about the pregnancy and her desire for an abortion, he said "whatever I decided to do, he was with me." Within a couple weeks, she found a clinic and made an appointment, relieved to learn that her insurance would cover the abortion. As was her regular practice, Valencia prayed to her god during this time. She believed that her religion considered abortion wrong and so asked her god for a sign of what she should do. She preferred not to disclose the signs she received to me in our interview but explained that "all of the signs that I was getting was pointing to not to have an abortion." Her language was specific: the signs related to not having an abortion; they did not tell her she should have another baby.

Valencia felt conflicted. She could not figure out how she and her husband could support another child, but she felt compelled to listen to the signs she had received. Still, she continued to think about abortion. Her body felt physically strained by this pregnancy, and she was struggling to carry the emotional responsibility for her entire family's well-being. She said she felt "a little overwhelmed because it's my body at thirty-five trying to carry a baby and having to worry about all these long-time goals instead of just the short term." She thought having an abortion would be the smart thing to do, but continuing the pregnancy felt like the morally right thing to do, after hearing from God: "The right thing to do would be to not have it—I mean to not go through with the abortion—to just have the baby. And the smart thing to do would be to think about the kids that I already have to worry about and terminate the pregnancy." Her decision making was focused on whether she could choose abortion, with recognition that not having an abortion would mean having a baby.

She talked to her husband and her mother about her decision and the signs she had received. She hoped her mother would support her choosing abortion: "She could have put the actual nudge in my back for me to make a smarter decision [of choosing abortion]." Instead, upon learning of the signs Valencia identified, both her mother and her husband articulated strong opposition to abortion: "Everybody was pretty much telling me not to do an abortion." Her loved ones insisted to her that God would not give her these signs unless his will was clear. Valencia's loved ones, in this way, also asserted that abortion was unchooseable.

Valencia went to the abortion appointment anyway and received medication abortion pills, but she did not take them at the clinic. Instead, she returned home and put them in her medicine cabinet. She gave herself a week to take the pills, but never did. During that time, she envisioned a certainty that choosing abortion would have karmic consequences. She said, "I had this overwhelming feeling that if I did go through with it that it would be bringing down a sense of something devastating to me that I wouldn't be able to handle." Believing that the stakes of her pregnancy decision were high, and with the means to terminate her pregnancy available, Valencia explained, "I really couldn't think of any reasons why [to have the abortion]." She had no affirmative reasons for continuing the pregnancy either, but that consideration had no relevance when abortion was unchooseable. Valencia felt that her reasons for abortion were insufficient compared to her reasons against abortion, which included opposition to abortion from loved ones and her evaluation that her god was opposed to her choosing abortion.

When Valencia and I spoke, the medication abortion pills sat in a drawer somewhere in her house. She was not planning to take them. She was not excited about having a new baby, either. As she explained, mostly she felt nothing about her pregnancy: "It's kind of weird. I feel like I'm going through a normal day. I just haven't really thought about too much other than sometimes you feel joy just being pregnant. I don't feel that. Sometimes you feel depressed about being pregnant. I can't really say I feel depressed. I don't really feel nothing about it." She hoped this dull feeling—a feeling notably different than the happiness she felt with the pregnancies for her four children—would not persist after the baby was born: "I feel like I'm just trying to cope with this pregnancy, and at the same time, trying to get through the next part and have the baby and not feel the same way I feel now being pregnant after I have the baby." Belief in the cultural narrative of abortion as against God's wishes stymied Valencia's ability to choose abortion, and it did not inspire attachment to her pregnancy. Her beliefs about abortion prevented her from having one, but they did not simultaneously affect her feelings about having a baby. In respondents' lives, antiabortion cultural narratives centering the fetus operated only on actions and feelings about abortion; they did not shape women's experience of attachment to their pregnancy.

Conclusion

A social understanding of abortion rooted in antiabortion activism that centered the fetus and potential life dominated the accounts of many respondents, in both Louisiana and Maryland. The construction of abortion as killing or against God's will changed the way the women described in this chapter engaged with pregnancy decision making. In practice, these narratives made abortion unchooseable.

Unlike the women described in the previous chapter, few of these respondents faced structural barriers to abortion. Indeed, those who did seek abortion care, like Aliyah and Valencia, did not face any structural barriers, and women like Kendra and Rashida had previous experiences of safe and accessible abortion. And yet, their decision making about abortion for this pregnancy was not unfettered. Abortion was unchooseable under the social meaning for abortion currently available to them. The upshot was that, despite not wanting to have a(nother) baby, they could not choose abortion. These cultural narratives operated as a barrier to abortion.

The experiences of the women whose accounts are discussed in this chapter illustrate the reach of antiabortion frameworks beyond restrictive policies. Abortion was unchooseable because of anti-abortion movement successes in framing the cultural meaning of abortion and, potentially, because of the lack of alternative reso-nant narratives. These women lacked access to cultural narratives that validated their consideration of abortion and constructed meanings for choosing abortion that were compatible with their sense of themselves as good people. Their experiences demonstrate that antiabortion advocates have been effective in propagating meanings for abortion that make it difficult for individual women like these respondents to choose abortion.

It is imperative to underscore that people who believe in fetal personhood, that abortion is killing, or that abortion is against God's will do still have abortions (Foster, Gould, et al. 2012; Jerman, Jones, and Onda 2016). Abortion patients are ideologically and religiously diverse. They are not required to believe that abor-tion is moral in order to receive abortion care. Likewise, belief in fetal personhood is not inherently antiabortion. Feminist scholars have advocated for an approach to determining fetal personhood that centers the determination of people with social relations to the fetus, such as the pregnant person and their partner, and the embodied experience of pregnancy (Layne 2003; Petchesky 1984). In its antiabortion iteration as inherent and absolute, however, fetal personhood diminishes the value of the pregnant person's deter-mination. Like structural obstacles, these cultural narratives oper-ate differently in different people's lives, sometimes becoming barriers to abortion. While these data cannot exhaustively point to when antiabortion narratives matter or for whom, this chapter illustrates how antiabortion narratives of the fetus can—and do—matter for some women who consider abortion.

Given patterning in rates of becoming pregnant when one does not want to be, and how race and class inequality undergirds this phenomenon, we should be attentive to how the operation of these narratives may disproportionately impact some populations. This potential impact is twofold. As this chapter has demonstrated, those who are pregnant when they do not want to be may be subject to cultural narratives that make abortion more difficult to choose. As a second effect, to the extent that these narratives make abortion unchooseable, they also reduce autonomy in choosing when to parent. That is, they represent a loss of autonomy about whether to have a baby as well as a loss of autonomy over when.

In the next chapter, I turn to cultural narratives in respondents' accounts that focused on the pregnant person (rather than the fetus), showing how they likewise could render abortion unchooseable. As with the narratives discussed in this chapter, I find that these pervasive cultural narratives have their origins in the anti-abortion movement.

4

Seeing Irresponsibility and Harm

As respondents considered abortion, they encountered a second kind of cultural narrative about abortion: narratives about the people who choose abortion. The pregnant people in these narratives were not, it bears clarifying, diverse, varied, and equally valued. Rather, the person in these narratives was the imagined, generic, monolithic, and gendered "woman." Far from attending to the specifics of her social location, these narratives constructed the imagined woman considering abortion in accordance with normative gender ideals of women as innately vulnerable and maternal and, simultaneously, as responsible for reproductive labor. As Tara's account illustrates, these constructed meanings could matter for respondents' ability to choose abortion.

Tara, a twenty-one-year-old Black woman in Maryland, felt upset when she discovered she was pregnant. Already stretched thin trying to provide for her two-year-old, Tara "didn't expect that [pregnancy] to happen," especially as she and her boyfriend of two years had been using condoms. As she explained, "I wasn't really ready for another child to be born in this world when I'm not really financially stable." She was also upset because she recognized that not continuing this pregnancy would mean choosing abortion—and she did not want to have to do that. She said, "I didn't know what to do, because I really don't believe in abortion." Like many of the respondents discussed in chapter 3, Tara subscribed to a narrative of abortion as killing, understanding abortion as "killing another child and stuff like that, even though I wasn't far [enough] along to say it was a child, but it's just like, it's growing inside of you." But there was more to her experience.

Tara also talked about abortion in terms of her feelings about sexual responsibility. Although Tara and her boyfriend had used condoms, she nonetheless asserted that by choosing to have sex, she had accepted responsibility for continuing any ensuing pregnancy. She said, "If you lay down and have sex with your partner, and you end up being pregnant, you shouldn't kill a baby, because of the simple fact that you could've wore a condom to prevent that. You could've had birth control maybe to prevent it, stuff like that." In Tara's logic, by willingly having sex and failing to prevent the pregnancy—even as she and her partner had used contraception—she was responsible for continuing it. Continuing a pregnancy was the responsible thing to do.

In addition, Tara told me that she believed obtaining an abortion would cause mental health harms. She said that, after abortion, "some people have depression. Some people have went killing theirself because they had to do it because [of] their living arrangements or somebody told them to and stuff like that." Tara did not know anyone who had had an abortion, let alone experienced depression or attempted suicide following an abortion. Nonetheless, she was confident that her belief was rooted in fact. She explained, "I have been reading on the Google, and they had a lot of stuff on where people [had abortions and] they went depressed and all that other stuff and ended up killing theirself. That stuff can happen." Her information was inaccurate (Biggs, Upadhyay, et al. 2017); abortion is not associated with increased anxiety or clinical depression. But Tara did not know that. Projecting this misinformation onto herself, Tara felt certain that she would have experienced depression after an abortion, saying, "I would've been very depressed, yes, I know I would've."

Immersed in these ideas about what choosing abortion would mean about and for her, but simultaneously clear that she did not want to be pregnant, Tara took no action related to her pregnancy for several weeks. Her boyfriend and the two friends she disclosed her pregnancy to said they were against Tara choosing abortion. She talked to her mom about the pregnancy, and her mom supported her choosing abortion, "but she said it's my decision, do what you want and stuff like that," offering only tepid engagement in Tara's decision making. Tara did not find talking to her mom about her pregnancy decision making helpful. For Tara, the opposition to and lukewarm support for abortion she encountered did not so much shift her thinking about abortion as curtail it. Tara could not find anyone to help her make sense of her strong desire not to be pregnant. In that absence, the meanings for abortion that were available to her—of abortion as killing, as irresponsible, and as causing depression—made actually choosing abortion hard to fathom.

In Tara's account, two common narratives about the meaning of choosing abortion are featured: abortion as sexually irresponsible and abortion as harmful to women. Tara was not the only respondent to think about abortion in these terms nor was she the only respondent for whom these narratives made abortion unchooseable. Like the meanings for abortion that center the fetus (see chapter 3), the proliferation and ubiquity of these meanings owe to the antiabortion movement. These narratives became barriers to abortion, mattering for women's ability to choose abortion, often without them ever seeking abortion care.

Abortion as Sexually Irresponsible

To examine the construction and influence of these cultural narratives of the meaning of choosing abortion, I start with one part of what made abortion unchooseable for Tara: her understanding that choosing abortion was avoiding her sexual responsibility (see also Edin and Kefalas 2011 for operation of this narrative in poor women's accounts of becoming single mothers). Another respondent in Maryland, Ebony, a thirty-year-old Black woman, applied a similar logic to her pregnancy decision making. Ebony discovered her pregnancy before she had even missed a period, when she was at the doctor's office to get contraception. They gave her a pregnancy test, and the results were positive. Stunned, as she put it, Ebony told me, "I didn't believe it, so I went home and bought my own [test]. Wasted money. But, yeah, that's what I did. I wasted money." With two positive test results, Ebony accepted the fact that she was pregnant. Initially, she was uncertain whether she wanted to continue the pregnancy. It was, she explained, unplanned, and she already struggled to support her two existing children as a single parent. She expected more of the same if she continued this pregnancy: "I know how hard it is to take care of two kids already, without the dad. And it's a guarantee that I'll be doing it for my third child. And I know for a fact it's going to be stressful." She knew this man was not likely to be an involved father—and she preferred that. She did not want to be tied to this man. Sometimes she felt he was trying to control her. Broadly, she explained, he represented "negative drama" she did not want in her life.

Still, Ebony found the idea of choosing abortion difficult. Part of her understood it as the best outcome for this pregnancy, and part of her felt obligated to continue the pregnancy out of a sense of sexual responsibility. As she put it: "I feel half-and-half about the situation. Half of me wants to go ahead, do what's the best for me [and have an abortion], and the other half says 'You knew what you was doing when you was laying down having that sex, that this could be a possibility.'" Ebony felt that choosing abortion was irresponsible, given that she had willingly had sex. In effect, she equated consent to sex with consent to parent. Because she had failed to "get on" contraception (presumably female body–based) earlier, she reasoned, this was something she brought upon herself. In this calculation, Ebony's autonomy to choose the circumstances under which she would have another baby ended when she consented to sex.

Chanel, a twenty-eight-year-old Black woman in Maryland, recounted a similar thought process. Chanel did not want to be pregnant. It did not feel like the right time. She waited two weeks after discovering her pregnancy before telling anyone about it, mostly ignoring it. As she said, "I wasn't thinking about that [the pregnancy] much." Choosing abortion, however, felt too difficult.

She explained, "I went back and forth with myself a few times like to go and get an abortion. I just didn't ever go. I couldn't. I couldn't do it. Because to me it's just like if you're woman enough to let it happen, you're woman enough to take care of your responsibility, and that's what I stick to." For Chanel, allowing pregnancy to happen—in the form of nonaction, by not taking action to prevent it—engendered an obligation to parent. In other words, her lack of action compelled future action and responsibility. Still, Chanel told me she considered abortion on and off for the entire first trimester of her pregnancy. Although, at the time of our interview, she was resigned to the fact that she could not choose abortion and would therefore be continuing her pregnancy, she was unenthusiastic about it. When we spoke, she was seventeen weeks pregnant and had not told anyone other than her boyfriend about her pregnancy.

These women all explained to me that they found it effectively impossible to imagine choosing abortion because they saw their pregnancies as the unsurprising outcome of decisions they had willingly made—that is, to have sex. And the responsible outcome of pregnancies, they reasoned, was birth and parenting, regardless of whether they wanted to parent under these circumstances. Abortion was unchooseable under this narrative. Their thinking about responsibility was gendered as well. While several spoke of the responsibility they had for becoming pregnant and for their pregnancy going forward, none spoke about the men they had sex with being responsible for the pregnancy (or for failing to prevent it), nor did they expect these men would play an active role in childrearing. Indeed, Ebony hoped the man involved would not continue to be in her life.

Shaunice's abortion decision making was influenced by related ideas about sexual responsibility. Shaunice, a twenty-one-year-old Black woman in Louisiana, had a one-year-old who had spent several days in the neonatal intensive care unit after she was born. The pregnancy had been exceedingly difficult for Shaunice and culminated in a traumatic labor experience during which she was close to having a seizure. She did not want to repeat that experience, at least not anytime soon. She had also recently started at a new job in food service that she loved—and that paid better and offered more hours than her prior employment. When she became pregnant, however, she had an extreme aversion to the smells at her new job. She would vomit the moment she entered her workplace. She would have to leave the job if she continued her pregnancy. She considered abortion: it was not the right time for another pregnancy and she did not want to lose this job. She said, "[I thought about abortion] because I had just got this great job, and I was making a lot more money, and then I couldn't stay. Like, that—that hurt."

When she brought up the idea of abortion to her husband, he quickly shut down the conversation. With no elaboration, she recounted, he objected to abortion. She told me, "He has no explanation [for opposing abortion]. It's just: 'We made the baby. Now be responsible.' That's just it." According to Shaunice's account of the conversation, after acknowledging his role in conception, her husband subtly shifted responsibility to Shaunice by using the command form of "be responsible." In his few words on the subject, he conveyed the expectation that it was Shaunice who was responsible for being responsible, and that abortion was not responsible behavior. Abortion was, in other words, not an option. He would not discuss it further.

Shaunice's mother would not talk with her about considering abortion either, saying, as Shaunice related, "'I never aborted any of y'all. I had all of my babies. And there was plenty of jobs I wanted to keep [but] I couldn't keep because I got pregnant.'" Shaunice's mother held her own behavior—that is, of "never abort[ing]"—as the appropriate standard, implying that deviating from this model was wrong.

Abortion still felt like the right choice for Shaunice. She turned to the Internet to try and sort out her thinking. She found a website that was explicit in its opposition to abortion: "It made a statement that it was going to teach you about abortion, but it, like, popped up and it told you, like, why abortion was wrong." She clicked through the slideshow on its homepage about fetal development that presented the fetus as a person. As Shaunice summarized, "it was just telling you, like, all the time that it takes to get an abortion, this living being is growing." This idea of fetal personhood and abortion as killing resonated with Shaunice, intersecting with her understanding of abortion as irresponsible. Given this context of fetal personhood, Shaunice explained, choosing abortion became selfish. She said, "I read through the entire thing [website]. And I knew all of those things, but [I was] just being selfish." She told me it was then that she realized abortion was not an option she could choose. The meanings for abortion available to her rendered abortion unchooseable.

THE CONTOURS OF THE ABORTION
AS IRRESPONSIBLE NARRATIVE

Ebony, Chanel, Shaunice, and Tara understood the meaning of abortion through a cultural narrative I term the "abortion as irresponsible" narrative. This narrative prescribed appropriate behavior for women, both before and after conception, and negatively judged deviations from that behavior. Women were expected to manage their fertility and prevent pregnancy when they did not want to have a baby. Respondents constructed pregnancy as a known and accepted consequence of people's sexual behavior and choices, a consequence that could be easily avoided by not having (unprotected) sex. Morgan, a twenty-seven-year-old Black woman in Maryland, for example, explained that "people know the choices that could happen [i.e., pregnancy] when they decide to do grown people things." Trinity, a twenty-three-year-old Black woman in Maryland, similarly, asserted that having sex without contraception meant accepting the possibility of (more) children: "When you lie down and have sex with people, think about that you don't need more kids. Think about how you can't take care of them before you lay down and have unprotected sex."

Generally, responsibility throughout this narrative was feminized. It was women who were responsible for managing fertility. Sometimes this feminization of responsibility was offered as a practical assessment, based in experience of men not taking responsibility. For example, Rashida, from chapter 3, said, "I feel like if people don't want to get pregnant, either get your tubes tied, get some type of birth control. . . . I just feel like if that's not what you want, then you should protect yourself at all times. Because the man won't do it and won't care about it." In other words, women had to take these actions because men would not. Other respondents feminized responsibility for pregnancy prevention unilaterally. Selena, a twenty-five-year-old Black woman in Maryland, explained: "It's the mom, their responsibility to wrap up or don't have sex at all. If you know that this can happen. I mean, they just set their self up." Pregnancy, in this logic, is constructed as the outcome of a failure to take sexual responsibility. Elsewhere during our interview, Selena said, "It's [pregnancy is] something that you know about and know that can happen. So, it's kind of like a consequence." Scholars have written about the unequal gendered division of fertility work, noting that women assume the greater share of physical, mental, and emotional responsibility for reproductive labor in heterosexual relationships (Bertotti 2013; Fennell 2011; Kimport 2018a; Littlejohn 2021). In U.S. culture, responsibility for preventing pregnancy is feminized.

This narrative constructed people who obtain abortions as shirking their reproductive responsibilities. Along these lines, Kara, from chapter 2, was concise, saying of getting pregnant, "It's not the baby's fault and you have to take responsibility for it." In this cultural narrative of sexual responsibility, when a woman fails to prevent a pregnancy, ending the pregnancy becomes a refusal to accept the consequences of her behavior. As Shaunice voiced, choosing abortion is selfish and irresponsible. Others echoed this theme. Trinity described people she knew who had abortions as "young and irresponsible." Jade, a twenty-nine-year-old Black woman in Louisiana, in response to a question about what kind of people she thinks have abortions, stated, "I would say selfish women. I don't know. I guess I would say selfish and maybe women that have been raped and things like that." For Jade, in other words, there were two categories of abortion patient: those who were selfish and those whose pregnancies were coerced. In response to the same question, Courtney, from chapter 3, told me that "people that's just out there and just not protecting themselves get abortions." Abortion is an outcome for people who fail to protect themselves—that is, fail to take responsibility for their sexual actions both before conception and after. Courtney elaborated that, further, certain people simply don't get abortions: "Not people that's been in relationships or, you know, building something. They don't get abortions." This cultural narrative positioned abortion as something irresponsible people choose, projecting certain qualities onto abortion recipients' character. Responsible people, it held, don't choose abortion.

More respondents from Louisiana than from Maryland negatively characterized women who obtain abortions, perhaps because more Maryland respondents reported knowing someone who had an abortion and more Maryland respondents themselves had a history of abortion, thereby rooting their ideas about abortion patients in real people. Knowing someone who had an abortion, however, was not always sufficient to combat this cultural narrative of people who get abortions as irresponsible. The construction of abortion patients as selfish could persist even when respondents knew and sympathized with someone who had an abortion. Mercedes, from chapter 2, for example, responded to a question about who gets abortions by saying: "Women who don't have morals, or just people that are actually not ready for it. But selfish—I mean, I don't know. I can't say, you know, because my friend [who had an abortion], she's not selfish. She's just being herself, she wasn't ready." This narrative of what it means to choose abortion broadly overwrote Mercedes's own perception of the people in her life who she knew had obtained abortions, pointing to its cultural salience and potency.

THE ROLE OF THE ANTIABORTION MOVEMENT

The idea that becoming pregnant carries with it a responsibility to parent is part of a longer history of contention over the role of women in society. Movements for and against abortion in the 1970s and early 1980s were characterized by different worldviews on gender, specifically on the place and responsibilities of women (Ginsburg 1998; Luker 1984). The antiabortion movement endorsed an understanding of gender premised on women as innately pro-spective mothers, constructing motherhood as not only natural but also as the only true fulfillment for women. Choosing abortion was a denial of women's nature and called into question their person-hood. When women are understood as essentially mothers, women who have abortions are marked as deviant. As anthropologist Faye Ginsburg (1998, 9) outlined in her classic book on prolife activists in the 1980s, a key premise of prolife activism was what she terms "antagonism to 'irresponsible sexual behavior.'" Irresponsible sex-ual behavior included having sex without the intention of procre-ation and failing to prevent pregnancy when pregnancy was not wanted. Pointedly, this behavior was understood to be natural to men but unnatural to women, thereby both gendering sexual behaviors and marking as deviant people who do not conform to these gendered expectations.

Abortion, under this logic, represents the ability to avoid the consequences for such "irresponsible sexual behavior." And thus, refusal of abortion represents taking responsibility after the fact for one's "irresponsible" behavior. Contemporary antiabortion activists, especially in the pregnancy help movement (also called the crisis pregnancy center movement), have continued to forward this construction of gender, emphasizing the importance of moth-erhood and normative gender roles in their opposition to abortion (Ehrlich and Doan 2019; Kelly 2012). In essence, this idea conflates sex (female) with role (parent/mother) (see also Doan and Schwarz 2020). In this way, it furthers normative gender, marking particu-lar behaviors as definitional of proper womanhood (i.e., continu-ing a pregnancy), and variations on that behavior (i.e., abortion) as deviant.

THE CHALLENGES OF "RESPONSIBILITY"

The ability to prevent pregnancy is more difficult than this narra-tive posits. Despite contention from Pamela, a thirty-one-year-old Black woman in Maryland, that "it takes nothing to go and protect yourself so you don't get pregnant," many women find it difficult to find and continuously use a method of contraception they like.

Most contraceptive methods have side effects that may interfere with everyday life as well as with the pleasurable experiences of sex (Higgins and Smith 2016). The literature has shown high rates of dissatisfaction with contraceptive methods, and these rates of dissatisfaction are patterned by education, with less-educated women more likely to be dissatisfied (Littlejohn 2012). Epidemiologist Lauren Lessard and colleagues (2012) surveyed women at high risk of unintended pregnancy about the features they would like in a contraceptive method (e.g., high efficacy in preventing pregnancy). They found that no currently available method of contraception has all their participants' highest ranked features. No existing method, in other words, meets all of women's preferences. A separate analysis of the same dataset by physician-researcher Andrea Jackson and colleagues (2016) demonstrated that women of color's preferences are least met by available, high-efficacy contraceptive methods. The decision to use a contraceptive method inherently requires accepting trade-offs.

And in heterosexual relationships, it is women who have to make these trade-offs. While this feminization is partly due to biotechnology, in that there are few contraceptive methods that operate in male bodies, it is nonetheless fundamentally socially constructed. In research (Daniels 2008), clinical interactions (Kimport 2018b), and romantic and family relationships (Fennell 2011; Littlejohn 2021), responsibility for preventing pregnancy is feminized. It is women who have to choose between contraceptive methods that have side effects and do not meet all of their preferences—or choose not to use a method at all. Further, to the extent that lower-efficacy methods have more of the features women of color prefer in a contraceptive method (Jackson et al. 2016), even among regular users of their preferred method(s), women of color may have more difficulty preventing pregnancy.

Normative ideas about pregnancy prevention also overlook patterning in who has access to their desired forms of contraception, including how healthcare systems and providers affect access (Dehlendorf et al. 2010; see also chapter 3). Low-income women and women of color are more likely to be uninsured than their higher-income and white counterparts, and may therefore have greater difficulty accessing contraceptive care and methods (Ebrahim et al. 2009). In their encounters with clinicians, low-income women and women of color are more likely to report feeling pressured into using a particular contraceptive method (Becker and Tsui 2008; Downing, LaVeist, and Bullock 2007; Mann et al. 2019) and to report experiencing race-based discrimination (Thorburn and Bogart 2005), both of which can reduce their interest in seeking contraceptive care and success in obtaining a method that meets their preferences.

Further, not using contraception can be an informed choice (Littlejohn 2021; Luker 1975). Even with the means and desire to prevent pregnancy, some people will choose not to do so, whether as a form of rejection of what sociologist Krystale Littlejohn (2021) terms compulsory gendered birth control or because it is simply too difficult (Luker 1975). After all, as public health scholars Jenny Higgins and Nicole Smith (2016) astutely recognize, people use contraception to have sex; they don't have sex in order to use contraception. Indeed, people who do not use contraception are not taking an unreasonable risk. In the absence of any contraceptive measures, the probability that a pregnancy will result from an act of unprotected vaginal sex is just 3 percent (A. Wilcox et al. 2001). Even this number misrepresents actual risk. As epidemiologist Allen Wilcox and colleagues (2001) found, for most of a menstrual cycle, there is almost zero risk of pregnancy. On the days around ovulation, the probability of pregnancy rises to as high as 9 percent, but this is still a relatively low risk of pregnancy. Even so, for some people, taking that chance will mean an unwanted pregnancy (Luker 1975).

In positing managing fertility as possible and expected, however, normative beliefs about sexual responsibility elide the feminization of reproductive labor and race- and class-associated discrepancies in access to contraceptive methods that meet patient preferences. Instead, they assert a narrative of individual responsibility, deflecting attention from social, provider-level, and health system factors that make avoiding pregnancy more difficult for some individuals. In addition, these normative beliefs tap into a loaded set of social meanings around "responsibility" as applied to people of color and low-income people. Women of color, especially Black women, are regularly portrayed in policy and media as financially, sexually, and morally irresponsible (Nadasen 2007; Rosenthal and Lobel 2016). In marking a particular course of action—that is, abortion—as "irresponsible," the abortion as irresponsible narrative intersects with extant social doubts about the responsibility of low-income Black women. The bifurcation between responsible and irresponsible behavior exists in a context wherein some people's actions are already more frequently constructed as irresponsible, but the narrative itself does not acknowledge this. Fundamentally, although there is no contraceptive method that is perfectly effective, and plenty of reasons why existing contraceptive methods do not work for all people who wish to avoid pregnancy, the responsibility narrative labels unplanned pregnancies as individual failures rather than the product of social structures, interactions, and a bit of chance.

Abortion Harms Women

The abortion as irresponsible narrative was not the only cultural narrative about people who choose abortion that influenced respondents' decision making. As Tara, from the opening of the chapter, referenced with her conviction that she would experience mental health harms from abortion, the narrative that abortion is harmful to women could make abortion unchooseable for respondents, even as scientific evidence disproves this claim (as I discuss below). Teresa, a twenty-six-year-old Black woman in Louisiana, is an example.

Teresa had just completed an associate's degree and intended to enroll in a four-year college when she discovered her pregnancy. For her, simply put, "it came at the wrong time." She had been planning to move to continue her schooling and worried that the pregnancy and parenting would compromise her ability to achieve her educational goals, especially living away from her mother.

Teresa told her mother she was considering abortion. In response, her mother warned her that abortion "might have a bad effect . . . like messing up the womb." Teresa understood this to mean that abortion could cause infertility. Neither Teresa nor her mother knew anyone who had experienced infertility following abortion, but Teresa trusted her mother's word. Although Teresa did not want to become a parent now, her desire to become a parent some-day and fear of losing that opportunity by having an abortion now meant she could not imagine choosing abortion. Because Teresa believed that abortion would make her infertile, abortion became unchooseable.

In the time since abortion became unchooseable, Teresa decided she could overcome any challenges having a baby posed for her life plans. At the time of our interview, she had moved in with her aunt while she sought to enroll at a four-year college, and her aunt had offered to help with the baby. As she summed up, "It was some-thing I realized I could live with. You know? It wasn't really a prob-lem afterwards." When abortion was not something she could choose, she adapted to the prospect of having a baby.

While Teresa's anticipated long-term physical harms because of abortion were different from Tara's anticipated mental health and emotional harms, both assumptions were rooted in an under-standing of abortion as a causal event with negative effects (see also chapter 5). They believed abortion harmed women—and would cause them harm. I term this narrative, consistent with other schol-ars' usage, the abortion as harmful narrative. Like the other cul-tural narratives I have discussed, the meanings for abortion this cultural narrative forwarded—of abortion as harmful—constrained respondents' ability to choose abortion. It differed from these other narratives, however, in that, aside from Teresa's case, it was more often a component of respondents' consideration than the single decisive factor impeding choosing abortion.

PHYSICAL HARMS

As in Teresa's account, many of the harms respondents expected abortion to cause were physical harms. In their conceptualizations, these physical harms were not the effect of an unskilled provider; they were an effect of abortion itself. For example, Kara, from chapter 2, avowed, "I know that abortion can be really damaging to the body," elaborating, upon prompting, that "[abortion can] affect the vaginal walls of some women [so] they're no longer fertile like they used to be." Khadijah, also from chapter 2, theorized a more detailed mechanism by which abortion causes physical harms. She said that abortion clinics should refuse to care for women who have multiple abortions, "because, in my eyes, I think you're creating a lot of scar tissue and a lot of problems with you." Nicole, a twenty-five-year-old Black woman in Maryland, conjectured that the harm of abortion is somehow related to the procedure. She said, "I think when you have surgical abortions, it does something [bad] to your organs on the inside." Even without a clear grasp on how abortion might cause physical harm, these respondents shared a general, unquestioned belief that abortion was harmful to women. Under this narrative, choosing abortion constituted taking a risk with one's physical health and future fertility.

They also, like Teresa, broadly lacked any personal experience of abortion causing physical harms. There were a few exceptions of tenuous experiential evidence. Trinity, for example, stated that she was opposed to "getting an abortion that can mess up my body" and later noted that her aunt was now unable to get pregnant when she wanted to be, years after having two abortions. Trinity suggested that it was the abortions that caused her aunt's current infertility, although she was unable to speculate how. Nicole similarly thought a history of abortion might be why a friend of hers was not pregnant, but she was not sure her friend wanted to become pregnant. She said, "I'm not sure if she can't conceive, actually. . . . I don't know if she's trying [to get pregnant] either." No other respondent could offer a real-life example of abortion causing physical harm.

The absence of evidence of abortion harming anyone they knew did not diminish respondents' faith in this narrative, signaling its cultural underpinnings. Indeed, the resonance of this narrative appeared to be impervious to empirical counterevidence. When I asked Teresa if learning that abortion does not cause future infertility would mean she might consider abortion for a future pregnancy, she answered in the negative, explaining that she doubted that could be true. She said, "I mean the thoughts of having it, it would trigger something. It would eventually trigger something."

MENTAL HEALTH AND EMOTIONAL HARMS

Like Tara from the opening of the chapter, other respondents imagined that mental health or emotional harms would ensue from an abortion. They anticipated emotional difficulty, regret, and sadness following an abortion. Deirdre, a thirty-year-old Black woman in Maryland, for instance, explained her belief that abortion inevitably causes difficult emotions, saying, "I'm sure anybody who has gotten an abortion before, even if they try to hide it that they didn't feel . . . a certain way about it, I'm sure they did."

Often, respondents' articulated expectations about the mental health and emotional harms of abortion stemmed from exposure to someone who had experienced postabortion emotional difficulty. For instance, Mercedes, from chapter 2, reflected that hearing stories from people who had abortions affected her own thinking about abortion. In particular, she referenced her best friend's emotionally difficult experience of abortion, saying, "I saw how it affected my best friend, where she still cries about it, and she tells me how she feels about it, sometimes crying. Especially when I told her that I was pregnant, she felt so overwhelmed and like, she was hurting on the inside, because she knew it was too late for her herself, you know. And it just made me feel like I can't go through that procedure." Several other women in Louisiana likewise reported knowing someone who had a bad emotional experience of abortion. Jade, from above, described going to an antiabortion pregnancy resource center years prior and hearing a presentation from a woman who regretted having an abortion. Jade explained that the speaker said "it [the abortion] haunted her for—for a long time, and she would hear a baby crying a lot. She didn't know where it was coming from. There wasn't a baby around her.

Just different little stuff that would haunt her." Shaunice also described hearing a presentation years ago—this one at a school event—during which the speaker talked about a prior abortion as "traumatic." This kind of public testimonial is a tactic of the anti-abortion movement (Ehrlich and Doan 2019; Haugeberg 2017; Kelly 2014). Other respondents knew someone personally who expressed emotional difficulty after an abortion. A friend of Camille's, from chapter 2, told her that her abortion "was not a good affair. She said she felt like she died. She said sometimes she'll still dream about her baby." Camille was hazy on the details because her friend shared the story many years ago, and they were no longer in touch. What remained, though, was Camille's awareness of the cultural narrative of abortion as causing emotional harm to women.

Among Maryland respondents, reports of knowing someone who had experienced emotional harm from abortion were fewer. For example, Kendra, from chapter 3, who had seven children, shared that several of her friends had abortions when they were younger. Now that they are older, she said, "they talk about it, I listen to what they say. They wish they never had abortions. And they kind of, like, give me a pat on my back because I kept, like, so many kids or whatever." Trinity related that her close friend had two abortions and told Trinity that afterward "'I hate[d] myself for a while.'" Trinity understood this to signify that her friend experienced negative feelings and even regret for having chosen abortion. She elaborated that although both of her friend's pregnancies were "with a guy she didn't want to be with, she really wished that she would have kept the babies." Few other Maryland respondents relayed knowledge of others having postabortion emotional difficulty. As I discuss in the next chapter, their personal experiences of abortion sometimes included postabortion emotional difficulty. While those experiences were consistent with this cultural narrative of abortion as causing emotional harm, I analyze them in the next chapter because respondents largely drew on them as a way to make sense of their embodied experience of abortion, rather than as a cultural narrative to make sense of abortion.

As the examples from respondents in both states suggest, the purported harms of abortion that respondents had interpersonal knowledge of were emotional, not clinical. No respondent reported knowing anyone who attributed depression, anxiety, or another diagnosed mental health disorder to an abortion experience. Yet, as with the narrative's assertion that abortion causes infertility, the absence of knowing someone who had experienced a mental health harm from abortion did not challenge respondents' framing of abortion as something that is harmful to pregnant people. Notably as well, in all these cases, respondents attributed the emotional difficulty they observed to the abortion itself, and not to the circumstances under which the abortion took place. In prior work, I have shown that postabortion emotional difficulty can stem from loss of a romantic relationship and experiences of social disapproval for choosing abortion (Kimport 2012). That is, the social situation can contribute to emotional difficulty (Kimport, Foster, and Weitz 2011), but this narrative narrowly ascribed causality for all emotional outcomes to the abortion itself.

THE ROLE OF THE ANTIABORTION MOVEMENT

The narrative of abortion as harmful has specific antiabortion origins. Sociologist Kimberly Kelly (2014) identifies the historical emergence and subsequent amplification of the claim of emotional harms in the 1970s. The idea that abortion could cause emotional and mental health trauma, she shows, began as a grassroots interpretive effort used by volunteers in local antiabortion pregnancy resource centers. In the 1980s, this framing was honed in antiabortion publications supposedly authored by women harmed by abortion (Haugeberg 2017) and gained traction in conservative think tanks. By the 1990s, when the antiabortion movement was losing public support, activists worried that their claims were too fetus-centric and so fastened on the abortion harms women claim as a way to oppose abortion seemingly on behalf of the pregnant person (Ehrlich and Doan 2019). This strategic framing enabled the antiabortion movement to continue to oppose abortion but to do so in language that did not appear to privilege the fetus over the woman.

Instead, its opposition to abortion was framed as an effort to protect women (Siegel 2008). The cultural narrative that abortion causes harm to the people who choose it, in other words, has been produced and advanced in service of the antiabortion movement.

There is, however, no evidence that abortion broadly causes physical, mental health, or emotional harms. Abortion is exceedingly safe (National Academies of Sciences, Engineering and Medicine 2018). Public health scientist Ushma Upadhyay and colleagues show that the rate of major adverse events following an abortion is less than a quarter of 1 percent (Upadhyay, Desai, et al. 2015). The mortality rate is exceedingly low as well: less than 1 per 100,000 abortions results in death (Raymond et al. 2014). There is also no evidence that abortion causes infertility (Frank et al. 1993). (It is worth noting that common treatments for miscarriage are the same as abortion procedures, but there is no associated claim of miscarriage management causing future infertility, further illustrating the strategic deployment of this claim.)

Similarly, there is no evidence that abortion causes mental health disorders or broad emotional difficulty. Empirical research demonstrates no correlation between a history of abortion and mental health disorders (Steinberg, Becker, and Henderson 2011). And prospective research examining the effects of abortion over five years finds no evidence that abortion causes anxiety, decreased self-esteem, or depression, but does find that denial of a wanted abortion is associated with a short-term increase in anxiety (Biggs, Upadhyay, et al. 2017). Likewise, there is no evidence that abortion broadly causes negative emotional outcomes or that most—or even many—women regret their abortion decision (APA Task Force on Mental Health and Abortion 2008; Rocca, Kimport, Gould, and Foster 2013; Rocca, Kimport, Roberts, et al. 2015). Five years after an abortion, 95 percent of women report that abortion was the right decision (Rocca, Samari, et al. 2020).

Absent scientific support, the narrative of abortion as harmful to women has nevertheless gained purchase in public discourse. It undergirds—and is naturalized through—state-level legislation restricting abortion (Doan and Schwarz 2020) and is present in judicial decisions on abortion. Perhaps most famously, in the 2007 majority opinion in *Gonzales v. Carhart*, U.S. Supreme Court Justice Anthony Kennedy asserted, "It seems unexceptionable to conclude some women come to regret their choice to abort the infant life they once created and sustained." As legal scholar Reva Siegel (2008) has argued, this is an example of the politicized iteration of the abortion harms women narrative, forwarding restrictions on abortion under a protectionist rubric: prohibiting abortion protects women. Not only does this narrative make abortion seem unsafe and risky, it also leverages and perpetuates the construction of abortion as a causal event. It makes abortion something that can be implicated for far-reaching consequences, even as "abortion" as a word does not describe a singular experience (Weitz and Kimport 2012), let alone a singular medical procedure. The termination of pregnancy, after all, can take place through pills, aspiration, dilation and evacuation, and induction of labor, among other methods.

Further, like other antiabortion cultural narratives, the abortion as harmful narrative obscures structural inequalities. Women of color, for example, are more likely to experience infertility but less likely to receive medical treatment for infertility (Greil et al. 2011). Because of environmental racism, some populations of women of color are more likely to experience infertility and adverse pregnancy outcomes due to environmental harms, such as heightened chemical and toxic contaminants exposure (Silbergeld and Patrick 2005). Poverty, structural racism, and microaggressions, too, have demonstrable negative impacts on people's mental and emotional health (Adler and Newman 2002; Clark et al. 1999; Kessler, Mickelson, and Williams 1999) and may themselves increase the negative impact of environmental harms (Gee and Payne-Sturges 2004). Assertions of abortion as the causal factor in people's experiences of negative physical and/or mental health displace attention from racial and socioeconomic disparities in infertility and mental health that are produced through laws, institutions, and practices. They invite, in other words, a different attribution—and associated remedy—for physical and mental health experiences than attention to structural inequalities.

Finding abortion unchooseable did not mean that respondents easily adjusted to continuing their pregnancies and the prospect of parenting a(nother) child. For Faith, a 30-year-old Black woman in Maryland, the abortion as irresponsible narrative was consequential in her decision not to obtain an abortion, but afterward she still found herself without an attachment to her pregnancy. Two years ago, Faith left the workforce when her daughter was born. She had been hoping to return to work and enroll her daughter in daycare soon. This pregnancy was unexpected. When she realized she was pregnant, Faith said, "I was just angry at myself, and you know, this wasn't really what I wanted, because I took the time off to stay home for two years with my daughter, so I decided that I wanted to go out to work, now that I did my job. And so now, I come to find out I'm pregnant again, it wasn't really the greatest news for me. It just made me feel a little down and upset." Faith chastised herself for being wrong about when she was fertile, blaming herself for the conception. She related that "all of me" felt like abortion was the right decision. Her fiancé agreed that this was not a good time for another baby. He had a long commute and worked long hours—and they still struggled to cover their rent. They needed a second income to cover their existing costs.

When Faith told her fiancé she thought abortion was the right decision for them, she told me, "he said the decision was mine." Her fiancé, in practice, abdicated any role in Faith choosing abortion as her pregnancy outcome. This was not what Faith wanted or expected. Usually, her fiancé spoke his mind and had opinions. In this instance, she did not want him to tell her what to do, but "I just needed confirmation." Faith needed her fiancé to agree with her choice, but he neither agreed nor disagreed. He declined to participate in the pregnancy decision making. Absent his articulated support for her decision, Faith did not feel that she could have an abortion. To do so would be irresponsible.

Without her fiancé's participation in the decision, Faith was at a crossroads. She did not feel that she could move forward with an abortion, but she felt no attachment to her pregnancy. She explained that "I'm just pretending like I'm not pregnant at this point." When I asked her what she thought her feelings about the pregnancy would be in the near future, she said, "I don't know. I'm hoping it cheers up. I'm hoping I cheer up." They were delaying their wedding. "Now," she said, "is not a good time."

The underpinnings of the cultural narrative of abortion as irresponsible meant that without her fiancé's support, Faith found abortion unchooseable. By removing himself from the abortion decision making, his action had the counterintuitive effect that Faith then felt she had no ability to choose abortion. Faith described herself as "accepting" the pregnancy but feeling about it the same way she did when she first discovered it: that it was not what she wanted. Even as she continued the pregnancy, she did not feel attachment or happiness about this outcome.

Other respondents did come to feel attachment toward their pregnancies, but not because the cultural narratives compelled it. Near the end of our interview, Tara, from the start of this chapter, told me that she was now "fine" with continuing her pregnancy. She felt that she had come to terms with being financially unstable and having another child. Unexpectedly, family members had stepped up to offer her support in the form of childcare for her two-year-old and even giving her money every so often. This help made the prospect of raising another child less daunting. Tara's feelings, it should be noted, emerged after she decided not to have an abortion; they were not why she opted to continue the pregnancy but rather a response—perhaps an adaptation—to that outcome.

Conclusion

As I have shown in this chapter, antiabortion cultural narratives about the people who choose abortion were pervasive in respondents' accounts of the meaning of abortion. These narratives asserted particular effects and outcomes of abortion: choosing abortion signaled irresponsibility and risked physical, mental health, and emotional harms. The abortion as sexually irresponsible narrative, in particular, tapped into normative gender expectations and raced and classed constructions of the idea of "responsible" behavior. Both of these narratives made abortion unchooseable for some respondents. Certainly, women who consider abortion to be an irresponsible choice and/or who believe abortion will cause them harm obtain abortions (Berglas, Gould, et al. 2017; Cockrill and Nack 2013; Foster, Kimport, et al. 2013; Gelman et al. 2017; Nickerson, Manski, and Dennis 2014), but such narratives of the meaning of choosing abortion made abortion unchooseable for the women whose accounts are discussed in this chapter.

Because of the abortion as harmful narrative, Teresa understood choosing abortion to put her ability to ever have children at risk—and she wanted future children. Because of the abortion as irresponsible narrative, Shaunice felt that choosing abortion was selfish, and she did not think of herself as selfish. These narratives operated on respondents' consideration of abortion, leveraging race- and class-based inequalities and normative expectations of gender. Ultimately, they made abortion unchooseable. These women were not continuing their pregnancies because they wanted to have a baby; they were continuing their pregnancies because abortion was unchooseable. Indeed, several of the respondents discussed in this chapter reported feeling no attachment to their ongoing pregnancy even as they knew they could not choose abortion.

These narratives were similar in origin, construction, and effect to antiabortion cultural narratives about the fetus. In practice, these two sets of cultural narratives did the work of antiabortion activists, constructing meanings for abortion that could make abortion impossible to choose. And, similar to some of the women whose accounts were discussed in chapter 2, they often did so before these women presented for abortion care. This underscores the reach of opposition to abortion, revealing how antiabortion ideology can constrain the decision making of pregnant people who never contact an abortion care provider.

The narratives of the fetus and the people who choose abortion that I have examined in this and the prior chapter do not exhaustively capture all the social meanings respondents ascribed to abortion. They were, however, the most prevalent across the sample. The operation of these narratives helps explain another part of the puzzle this book grapples with of why women consider but do not obtain an abortion. In the face of antiabortion cultural narratives, abortion can become unchooseable, upending the assumption that all pregnant people have "choice" in the outcome of their pregnancy.

5

Fearing the Experience of Abortion

Structural obstacles and antiabortion cultural narratives accounted for much of why respondents considered and did not obtain an abortion. Those factors rendered abortion unchooseable for many of the women I interviewed. But some respondents' experiences remain unexplained. Pamela, a thirty-one-year-old Black woman in Maryland, is one of those women. When Pamela discovered her current pregnancy, she had recently broken up with her boyfriend. She explained, "We just had a huge falling out, and just decided we were never going to talk again." She was already raising two children as a single parent. The father of her twelve-year-old died when her daughter was two. Her two-year-old son's father is in his life, but Pamela still is the primary—and often sole—caregiver for him. She worried that this pregnancy represented another child she would have to raise alone. She told me of the prospect of being a single parent to a third child, "I just didn't want to do that because it's hard on kids." Pamela considered abortion.

This consideration took place alongside experiential knowledge of abortion. When Pamela was twenty-three, she had an abortion. It felt like the right decision at the time and still does to Pamela. A few years after that, she discovered she was pregnant and, again, felt it was not the right time to have a baby. She had an abortion, but this time it was different. Her relationship with the man involved—her two-year-old son's father—was emotionally complicated. They were in a rough patch, but she wanted to be with him. This made her experience of abortion emotionally different from her first abortion, and more difficult. She explained, "That [abortion] was the best thing for me. But afterwards it just took a toll on me emotionally. . . . Really screwed me up mentally. So, after that I was just kind of like, you know, I can't do that anymore." Like the vast majority of women who report negative emotions after an abortion (Rocca, Samari, et al. 2020), Pamela still felt that "ultimately, I know it was the right thing to do at the time." In prior work, I have shown how the relationship context in which an abortion takes place can be related to postabortion emotional difficulty (Kimport 2012; Kimport, Foster, and Weitz 2011). Pamela recognized how it was her complex romantic relationship that mattered for her postabortion emotional experience. But she was still wary that another abortion, even under different relationship circumstances, could have a similar emotional impact.

Wishing to avoid such an experience, she rethought breaking up with her boyfriend. She called her (ex-)boyfriend and told him about this pregnancy. He was surprised. Then, she said, they sat down and talked things through: "So, he took off from work, and we sat down and talked. And went out and got lunch. And just sat down and decided that we were going to, you know, give our relationship another shot. And he would move back in. And we would try to do things, you know, the right way for the baby. For the pregnancy." After Pamela and her boyfriend talked things through, she felt like she could make the relationship work and have a baby. She was relieved not to have another abortion.

Pamela considered abortion because she did not want to raise another child as a single parent. By getting back together with her boyfriend and getting his assurance that he was going to be an actively involved parent, she resolved this concern. What is important to highlight in her account is that underlying this sequence of events was a desire to avoid abortion. Pamela did not resume her romantic relationship because she wanted to have a baby. She reached out to her (ex-)boyfriend because she did not want to have another abortion, concerned that she would have a negative emotional response to abortion. This experience-informed anticipation constrained what it meant for Pamela to choose abortion, making abortion unchooseable regardless of her feelings about having a baby.

As it was for Pamela, abortion could become unchooseable for respondents who were not constrained by structural obstacles or cultural narratives based on their expectations about what the embodied experience of abortion would be. As described in chapter 1, I conceptualize embodiment to encompass physical and emotional experiences as well as perceptions, meaning making, and the self. For the women whose accounts are discussed in this chapter, embodiment was rooted in the social experience of physicality, across multiple dimensions. Often, like Pamela, respondents' expectations of what choosing abortion for this pregnancy would mean were informed by prior experiences of abortion. Among respondents without a history of abortion, their experiences and expectations of health care generally contributed to their sense of the embodiment of abortion.

In this chapter, I introduce the idea of "anticipated embodiment of abortion," showing how what respondents anticipated an abortion would be like could affect their pregnancy decision making, especially if they anticipated that an abortion experience would be negative physically or emotionally. This anticipated negative embodiment, like the structural and cultural barriers discussed in prior chapters, constrained respondents' ability to choose abortion and could render abortion unchooseable. I also introduce evidence of medical mistreatment of some respondents in their reproductive health care, which affected their use of health care and had consequences for their ability to manage their fertility. I close the chapter with the accounts of three respondents for whom anticipated negative embodiment of abortion informed their desire not to seek a clinic-based abortion and, instead, to attempt to end their pregnancy on their own.

Prior Experience of Abortion

In describing their consideration of abortion, several respondents discussed a prior experience of abortion and how it conditioned their ability to choose abortion for this pregnancy. Having a history of abortion was more common among Maryland respondents (see Methodological Appendix), so it is unsurprising that most of these women were in Maryland. For some, abortion was a physically difficult experience they did not want to repeat. Ebony, introduced in chapter 4, remembered her aspiration abortion ten years prior as her most painful reproductive experience—and she had given birth twice. As recounted in chapter 4, the cultural narrative of abortion as irresponsible was central to her abortion decision making. Her experiential knowledge of the embodied experience of abortion mattered as well. She explained of her abortion at age twenty, clarifying that her negative memory of abortion was specific to an aspiration—also sometimes called "surgical"—abortion: "I felt everything. And that was scary. And that traumatized me for a long time. So I would never do surgical, I would do the pills, and I know it's definitely too late for the pills. And I refuse to get surgical. Won't happen." Ebony discovered her pregnancy early enough to be eligible for a medication abortion (also known as abortion pills), which, at the time, was approved for use up to the tenth week of pregnancy. Her belief in the cultural narrative of choosing abortion as irresponsible slowed her decision making, initially making her feel unable to choose abortion. As that delay wore on, the window for medication abortion closed. With only aspiration procedures now available, abortion was unchooseable for Ebony.

For most other respondents with a history of abortion, however, what they sought to avoid was not so much the physical experience of abortion but what happened after the abortion. As alluded to in chapter 4, several described personal experiences of postabortion emotional difficulty, and this conditioned their embodied understanding of abortion. For instance, after obtaining an abortion the year before our interview, Deirdre, a thirty-year-old

Black woman in Maryland, faced antiabortion protesters outside the clinic. A religious Christian who goes to church weekly, she described this encounter and its effects on her: "They had the picture of Christ and the Bible and everything and it really made me really emotional." The abortion felt like the right decision at the time, but the confrontation with protesters citing antiabortion religious dictates made her feel bad. As research has shown, high perceived community abortion stigma is associated with postabortion negative emotions (Rocca, Samari, et al. 2020). While the protesters did not create Deirdre's negative association with abortion, their signs leveraged her existing internalized stigmatization of abortion. With her current pregnancy, Deirdre anticipated she would feel bad after another abortion. She thought of abortion as causing those bad feelings, not the antiabortion protesters or stigmatization of abortion. She did not think she could repeat that emotional experience. In practice, Deirdre associated the feeling of shame the antiabortion protesters prompted with choosing abortion, rendering abortion unchooseable for her current pregnancy.

Multiple respondents voiced concerns like Deirdre's about the emotional aftermath of abortion, including a set of several respondents who described being pressured into a prior abortion. Melissa, a twenty-six-year-old Black woman in Maryland, was one example. Melissa had an abortion when she was a teenager, but the decision did not feel like her own. Her guardian, she said, "basically drove me down to the clinic and paid in cash." Melissa said, "I didn't really have a choice but to go through with it." This felt bad to Melissa. In our interview, Melissa attributed this bad feeling not to the adult who pressured her but to the abortion itself, vowing never to obtain another abortion.

Similarly, Nicole, a twenty-five-year-old Black woman in Maryland, recalled a pregnancy when she was a teenager that she felt pressured to terminate. When Nicole became pregnant, her mother kicked her out of the house and suggested she get an abortion. Her boyfriend's reaction was stronger. She said, "My boyfriend at the time did not want me to have the child, and he threatened to kill me if I did." I asked her if she felt like this was something he would actually do: Did the threat feel real? She responded, "At the time, I wasn't sure. I don't take those type of threats lightly. I don't think that he's that type of person, but I just didn't want to take the chance, just in case." Nicole had an abortion and felt supported by her friends. Afterward, she said, she also felt "ashamed, bad, [and] disappointed in myself." She felt as though her decision to have an abortion was not her own. In reaction, she was determined not to have another abortion, believing that any future abortion would feel equally coerced. Her desires regarding having a baby and under what circumstances did not figure in this decision making. As I described in chapter 1, Nicole reported that the man involved in this pregnancy had been physically violent toward her, and she anticipated this would happen again.

Alexis, an eighteen-year-old Black woman in Maryland, is a final example of how a prior experience of being pressured into abortion could influence current thinking about abortion. Several months before her current pregnancy, Alexis had an abortion. She was in her senior year of high school, and her grandmother pressured her to terminate the pregnancy. Alexis related that her grandmother made her feel ashamed of being pregnant in her teens. Her grandmother, she said, "was just real negative. Everything about having a baby so young was just so negative. Like, everything [she] said out of [her] mouth was just negative, negative, negative, negative, negative. And it just put in my head, like, it was just so wrong [to have a baby then]." Alexis had an abortion and found it physically painful. Soon afterward, she felt emotionally off. She did not quite know how to explain it, saying, "I don't know, that's when I really, like, I don't know. I just was messed up off of that." She attributed her emotional reaction to the abortion itself. She promised herself she would never have another abortion.

When she discovered her current pregnancy, however, Alexis thought hard about obtaining an abortion, going so far as to schedule an abortion appointment. Alexis considered abortion, as first described in chapter 1, because she worried about "not finishing school or something, or being a young mother. Not being the best mother I could be, stuff like that." But as the abortion appointment approached, she could not shake off her memory of her prior abortion. Believing her negative emotions were tied to abortion itself rather than the circumstances under which it took place, Alexis told me she feared that having a second abortion would be "too much" for her to handle: she anticipated a negative postabortion emotional experience and so felt abortion was unchooseable. She did not show up to her abortion appointment.

As I detailed in chapter 4, scientific evidence refutes the claim that abortion causes mental health harms and that negative postabortion emotions predominate. In other work, I have shown that the social circumstances surrounding an abortion can contribute to postabortion emotional difficulty (Kimport, Foster, and Weitz 2011) and that emotional circumstances and aftermath can differ significantly between abortions for the same person (Weitz and Kimport 2012). Rather than the medical experience of abortion being the cause of difficulty, I argue, the social context in which the abortion takes place is of consequence. In making sense of their own lived experiences, nonetheless, respondents who reported a negative prior experience of abortion associated their bad feelings with abortion itself, not with the circumstances around their abortion. When abortion was understood as the cause of emotional difficulty, for women who did not want a negative embodied experience of abortion, it became unchooseable.

One respondent made a further attribution, believing that her prior abortion caused her to have an incompetent cervix in her subsequent pregnancies. By the time of our interview, Tandra, a thirty-four-year-old Black woman in Maryland, had a pregnancy history that included multiple miscarriages in the second trimester (which are far less common than first-trimester miscarriages), five births, and an incompetent cervix for her most recent three pregnancies. Tandra had a first-trimester abortion after her two oldest children were born and then experienced an incompetent cervix in the pregnancies for her three subsequent children. It made sense to her that the abortion was the cause "because I didn't have that problem prior to [the abortion]." There is no scientific data connecting abortion and incompetent cervix in subsequent pregnancy, but it made sense to Tandra. Her understanding of abortion was informed by her reproductive experiences. She also remembered her abortion, nearly ten years prior, as "really, really painful." She summed it up as "a horrible experience."

Tandra had requested a tubal ligation after the delivery of her youngest child, but at the time she went into labor, well before her due date, her paperwork was not complete. Women who receive Medicaid, like Tandra, are subject to a federal policy requiring that they complete sterilization paperwork at least thirty days before the procedure. Tandra therefore could not request a tubal ligation right when she went into labor. People with private insurance are not subject to this waiting period. Although the policy was intended to protect vulnerable populations, for women like Tandra, it meant she was unable to get her desired sterilization (see also Borrero et al. 2014). Then, about three months after her youngest was born, her period stopped, and she suspected she was pregnant. Having recently ended her relationship with the father of her newborn, at first Tandra ignored the pregnancy, "just hoping that my period would just come, but it didn't." She waited a few more weeks, busy with her new baby and existing children. She took a store-bought pregnancy test, which came out positive. Her first thought was that abortion was the right decision. As she said succinctly, abortion felt like the right decision because "I just had my daughter and [I'm] high-risk [in pregnancy] already and I knew I didn't want any more kids." The man involved in the pregnancy, her ex, said he would support her in whatever outcome she chose. She told her mother, aunt, and brother about the pregnancy and her consideration of abortion. Like her ex, they were all supportive of whatever outcome she chose, telling her they understood why she was considering abortion. Throughout these conversations, Tandra struggled to reconcile her desire not to have another baby with the fact that abortion felt unchooseable, given her belief that it caused health problems and her desire to avoid the physical pain she associated with abortion. At the time of our interview, Tandra was resigned to continuing her pregnancy but told me she hoped it would end in miscarriage, as had so many of her previous pregnancies.

In assigning to abortion the power to cause emotional difficulty and, in Tandra's case, bodily harms, these respondents elucidate the rhetorical availability of abortion for blame. As they sought to make sense of their embodied experience of abortion, these women assigned causal power to abortion, and deflected responsibility from the context in which their abortions took place. Rhetorician Nathan Stormer (2015) argues that the rhetorical frames for discussing abortion—and, particularly, the abortion rate—established by physicians in the nineteenth century have produced abortion as a stand-in for a range of social and moral concerns, forwarded by multiple and often competing facets of society. In contemporary debates, the abortion rate has taken on an evidentiary role for social phenomena not directly connected to clinical provision of abortion, from women's liberation to conservative family values.

I posit that we find evidence of a similar phenomenon in these accounts of how respondents made sense of their embodied history of abortion. They understood abortion as a causal event with effects that exceeded ending a pregnancy, interpreting the emotions around the physical experience and sometimes subsequent health problems as caused by abortion itself. Although there is no scientific evidence supporting these associations, with this embodied understanding of abortion, choosing abortion for this pregnancy became impossible.

Assessing the Conditions of Care

Anticipating a negative embodied experience of abortion, and finding abortion unchooseable because of it, did not depend on having a previous experience of abortion. Some respondents drew on their observations of available abortion care or knowledge of abortion from other sources and compared these to their expectations for care. For example, Madison, a 27-year-old white woman in Louisiana, had not had a prior abortion, but her initial visit to the local abortion clinic, per Louisiana's two-visit requirement, informed her thinking about what having an abortion would be like—and that anticipated negative embodiment made abortion unchooseable. Madison had struggled to find an abortion provider in Louisiana. She tried many tacks to get information about abortion, including searching the Internet and calling the local health information hotline, and was frustrated at every turn. In the end, none of these search efforts worked. She only found a clinic after disclosing her pregnancy to her roommate, who then told her about a local abortion clinic. She made an appointment.

Even with an appointment, the specifics of care at that clinic—partly conditioned by laws and partly by the clinic's service model—made abortion seem arduous. Madison identified time and scheduling burdens along with missed work and travel costs. On top of those logistical challenges, for Madison, after attending her first visit, this clinic in specific did not seem like a place she wanted to receive an abortion. For one, she thought some of their practices seemed unsanitary. She described the cleaning of the ultrasound equipment as perfunctory: "And I don't know what she was wiping it with, but then she just, like, puts it back on the machine, and, like, she's going to use that on the next girl. So, like, what are you actually sanitizing? And I don't know. Like, that just seemed really strange to me, and pretty gross." She felt put off by the physician as well, whom she described as arriving hours after all the patients had completed their paperwork. Madison thought this was unprofessional and, lacking any explanation from clinic staff about this timing, attributed the long day abortion patients had to undertake at the clinic to the physician's whims. Further, Madison did not like the physician's affect and found the music the physician played to be inappropriate. Of the clinic, Madison summarized: "It's unprofessional, and it makes me feel really uncomfortable. It, like, seems very unsanitary. And then, you have this woman who's supposed to be a doctor, and you're supposed to, like, respect this doctor to do this. And she's, like, telling you, like, 'You better not cry,' and she's playing rap music that's, like, cursing in the background. I mean, it's pretty bad." Rooted in specific observations, Madison conveyed a suspicion of abortion providers that is consistent with antiabortion efforts to stigmatize healthcare workers who provide abortions (Doan and Schwarz 2020; Freedman 2010; Joffe 1995; O'Donnell, Weitz, and Freedman 2011; Weitz and Kimport 2015). In this way, her critique of the clinic was connected to cultural narratives that foment distrust of abortion providers as well as to her anticipated embodied experience of abortion. During the counseling portion of the appointment, she learned that the clinic did not offer anesthesia, which Madison strongly wanted, and abortion became unchooseable for her.

Although abortion care is often conceptualized strictly as an outcome, it is useful to recognize that Madison sought not just an abortion, but an abortion with certain conditions of care. In effect, she was acting as a healthcare consumer. Because she was unable to find care under the conditions she desired at the clinic she found and unable to find a different provider, abortion was not chooseable for Madison. She re-evaluated her circumstances. The man involved in the pregnancy was a friend she had been casually seeing in recent months, a rebound relationship after ending a multiyear engagement. It was a time of significant personal change, and her family was worried about her adjusting to these changes. Although the man involved was clear that he did not want her to continue the pregnancy and these were not Madison's desired circumstances for becoming a parent, the conditions of the only abortion clinic she could find were decidedly not conditions under which Madison would have an abortion. And with abortion unchooseable, her resolve that abortion was the right decision began to fade. She rationalized that, six months prior, she had been looking forward to marrying and becoming a mother and, just because things had not gone as planned, why shouldn't she become a mother now? She explained, naturalizing the barriers she faced, "You know, and even though it's not ideal, my train of thought is, like, I'm close to thirty years old. I am capable, you know. I'm not a little girl, you know. And I'm really used to being around kids, so it just kind of seems, like, natural that I would keep it." Underneath this rationalization, however, her account shows that it was her experientially informed aversion to the only care provider she could find that made abortion unchooseable and led to her continuing her pregnancy.

Madison was not the only Louisiana respondent who had a negative opinion of a local clinic. Mercedes, from chapter 2, did, too. Months prior to her pregnancy, Mercedes accompanied her friend to an appointment there, aware that it was one of only two local clinics still open. She did not like what she saw. She said of the abortion clinic she visited, "I've been to one of them with my friend when she got her abortion, when she wanted me to go with her to her second appointment, and it's so disgusting. Everything's unsanitary." She anticipated that being in that space for an abortion appointment would make her unable to choose abortion. Referencing her knowledge that abortion appointments often require a great deal of waiting and counseling on the abortion decision, she explained, "If I would've had to sit there for three hours just to see the doctor to re-evaluate my decision, and looking at that place and how like raunchy it looked, I would probably not go all the way with it." Interestingly, she was not so much concerned with the experience of the counseling dissuading her from abortion as she believed that having to spend time in a space that did not meet her expectations for a medical care facility would make it impossible to choose abortion.

As detailed in chapter 2, Mercedes's story is more complicated than this. She reported that she and her boyfriend planned on abortion until her mother declined to give them the money for it and they realized they could not afford an abortion. Still, Mercedes's anticipation of what being in that specific clinic would be like was also part of her pregnancy decision making.

Another respondent without prior experience of abortion anticipated a negative embodied experience of abortion based on online research. April, a twenty-year-old Black woman in Louisiana, wanted to be older, married, and in a better romantic relationship before she had children. She and her partner had been off and on for two to three years. They argued a lot. April called these arguments "the usual struggles." When April discovered she was pregnant, she knew her mom would be upset. Her mom had big dreams for her: "She had like plans for me to like travel and everything like that." April thought about seeking an abortion, in part, because of

> my mom, the idea of not being able to travel and have this fantabulous movie life that I dreamed of. And the guy of course, I mean you know it's just like: I don't know if I want to do this. I don't know if I like you right now. We're not married. So, you know, wanting to wait until you're married to have a kid. That way you know that everything is set for the most part, as set as it can be. And so, like yeah, I worried about that. And I was just like, do I really want to do this [have a baby]?

April felt informed about her pregnancy options. She explained to me, "They're [pregnancy options are] always there, like from all the movies I've seen, from all the life experiences that I've had." Yet she also had practical questions. She did not know anyone who had an abortion and wondered, "How would you do it? How would you ask for it? How would you schedule it?" She knew about abortion as an idea but not as health care she could obtain.

April was in an information vacuum, and opposition from others in her life complicated her ability to gather information. When she told her partner she was considering abortion, he voiced opposition. Couching his opposition in deference to her as the person who was pregnant, April related, "he was like, 'It's your body, but I'm not supporting you.' . . . He said that, like, repeatedly because I spoke of it various times." She talked to a close friend about considering abortion, but the friend had little to offer her, telling her "just look it up."

April looked up the phone number of an abortion clinic and called them, but it was outside of business hours and she only got a recording. The recording did not answer her questions. April turned to the Internet. She explained, "I just decided to look up the procedure online. And I saw some videos." Online, April learned about gestational limits, the option of medication abortion, and that aspiration abortion works through suction. The idea of suction was disturbing to her. It made her think of abortion differently, anticipating negative embodiment. "I was just like, 'Oh, they're going to suck it out of me? Oh, what if it could be like a baby at this point?' I was like, 'Oh, nevermind.'" Although I did not see the websites April consulted, the information she reported learning from them was accurate, if incomplete. And this information contributed to what she anticipated her embodied experience of abortion would be, making it unchooseable for her.

April could imagine someone choosing abortion, summoning up the hypothetical pregnant person "who feels that this is the right choice for them, like a woman who is in like hardship, maybe, and, hopefully, just think it's the right decision for them. . . . I just think if it fits your situation because if it's the right decision, you should make it." In her assessment of her own pregnancy, however, abortion was unchooseable when she envisioned a suction abortion. She had no other sources of information about abortion, let alone about the embodied experience of abortion. She did, however, have access to antiabortion cultural narratives. April began to think of her developing fetus as an independent life and to reframe her circumstances as intended by God. She said, "I was like, I might as well just take this wonderful life as whatever it could be, and I don't know, it could be like the best thing that ever happened to me. Everything happens for a reason." In the absence of accurate information and social support for abortion, anticipating a negative embodied experience of abortion, April relied on the cultural narratives of abortion that were available to her, all of which were antiabortion. In this context, she reassessed her situation as "not terrible" and thus as not meeting the threshold for choosing abortion. She said, "I just decided, no, I'll just see what life has for me. I was like it's not terrible. I said, I don't have to have an abortion." And she called on herself to defer to God's plan, saying, "Got to see what life's put in front of me, what the Lord has put in front of me, and maybe just take it as another adventure."

Medical Mistreatment

My discussion so far in this chapter has focused on respondents' personal experiences of abortion, including their anticipated experiences. These were things the interviews covered in depth. Respondents also talked about other experiences of health care, many of which were poor. As I described in chapter 1, socially vulnerable populations have been underserved and mistreated by the healthcare system. Many respondents had personal experience of this. Absent personal experience, they had a general awareness of low-income patients receiving poor medical treatment and the existence of racial discrimination from providers. In several instances, previous experiences of poor health care contributed to their current pregnancy circumstances and could operate as a constraint on their ability to choose abortion.

Negative experiences of obtaining reproductive health care in the past, for example, including accounts of forced cesareans and other obstetrical violence, could have a direct bearing on respondents' ability to choose abortion for this pregnancy. In recounting her pregnancy history, Khadijah, from chapter 2, described obstetric violence. She told me, "I had three C-sections. My second one, I actually got scared into." Khadijah felt mistreated by her obstetric team, which contributed to a general distrust of medical professionals. Additionally, her history of multiple cesareans had implications for future pregnancies. People with a history of multiple or very recent cesareans face greater medical risk in abortion as the pregnancy progresses (as well as in labor and delivery for pregnancies carried to term), prompting some clinicians to advise patients seeking abortion later in pregnancy who have a history of cesareans to obtain care in an inpatient setting, with more medical support (American College of Obstetricians and Gynecologists 2013). As detailed in chapter 2, Khadijah was already into her second trimester when she discovered this pregnancy, and her history of cesareans, including the one she felt forced into, was therefore consequential to whether it was safe to care for her in an outpatient setting. Because of her history, the physician at the outpatient abortion clinic she visited declined to provide her abortion and, instead, referred her to a hospital for care.

Her past experience—and the distrust it engendered—had further implications for her current pregnancy. When she did find an abortion provider at a hospital, their practices around scheduling were strange to Khadijah: she thought it suspicious that they had a waiting list (see chapter 2). And although lack of transportation ultimately prevented her from obtaining an abortion, the hospital giving her only thirty minutes notice before an abortion appointment was available also seemed suspect. No one explained these practices to Khadijah, and, given her history of negative treatment in a hospital, she was not inclined to trust healthcare workers. Khadijah did not see the healthcare workers at the hospital as people who could help her obtain the abortion she wanted, and so did not convey her concerns and skepticism to them. Instead, she took herself off the waiting list for an abortion and resigned herself to being unable to choose abortion.

Previous experiences of health care mattered for other respondents' current pregnancy circumstances as well. Consistent with evidence of the stratified difficulty in preventing pregnancy (see chapter 4), some respondents' pregnancies themselves were the result of poor medical care—bordering on medical mistreatment—and/or distrust of the healthcare system. For instance, Deirdre was pregnant when she did not want to be because of poor medical care. Deirdre, who above described feeling shamed by antiabortion protesters after a previous abortion, had been using an intrauterine device (IUD) to prevent pregnancy for about a year, but it started to cause her pain. She went to the emergency room, and they discovered that the IUD had migrated out of the uterus. The clinician refused, however, to remove the IUD for her, telling her, "They [the emergency room staff] wouldn't take it out because they said they weren't the ones who put it in." Still in significant pain, Deirdre called several other hospitals until she found one that would remove the IUD. She had to wait two days for an appointment but finally got the IUD removed, and the pain disappeared. The clinician there offered her alternative contraception, but after her difficult experience trying to get the painful IUD removed, she did not trust either the healthcare system or the safety of other prescription contraception. When she discovered she was pregnant when she did not want to be a few months later, she was not surprised. In essence, Deirdre was pregnant because the inadequate and insensitive reproductive health care she received engendered medical mistrust.

Alexis, too, who felt pressured by her grandmother into a previous abortion, distrusted the healthcare system and prescription contraception, and this distrust impeded her ability to prevent pregnancy. Alexis did not use contraception because she was skeptical of its long-term safety. She told me: "Some women, if you're on birth control too long—which they will not tell you—you will not be able to have kids. Some young teens got to go through that or they die from birth control. I'd be scared. I don't want to be putting nothing in my body that might kill me in the future because I'm taking it too much, or prevent me from having other children because of these doctors trying to put so much medicine in you. I don't like that." She declined to share this with her doctor, however, simply telling the doctor that she did not use contraception because she did not want to. When I asked her why she did not elaborate with her physician, she said, "I didn't tell her that to her face because I didn't want her to feel bad." They did not have a relationship based on trust and open communication. Alexis's concerns about the harmful effects of contraception are not broadly supported by scientific evidence. Existing prescription contraceptive methods are safe for most bodies, but they do have side effects, and, in rare instances, some can cause adverse events, including death (World Health Organization Reproductive Health 2007). While there are some characteristics that are known to increase risk of adverse events, there is also uncertainty: physicians cannot predict who among those with no known risk factors will experience side effects or adverse events (World Health Organization Reproductive Health 2007). Further, as Alexis anticipated, sociologist Krystale Littlejohn and I (2017) have shown that clinicians who counsel patients on birth control tend to minimize, contest, or discount the risks individual patients face.

There is also historical precedent for a suspicion of prescription contraception and of delivery of contraception through the health-care system from a specifically women of color standpoint. As mentioned in chapter 1, women of color's desire to manage their fertility has been exploited in testing for contraceptives (Gordon 2002), and they have been subject to population control through sterilization without their consent (Nelson 2003; Roth and Ainsworth 2015; Schoen 2005; Stern 2005). Moreover, women of color themselves report being pressured by their provider to use partic-ular, usually non-patient-controlled forms of contraception (Down-ing, LaVeist, and Bullock 2007; Thorburn and Bogart 2005), which may or may not meet their preferences. In other words, there is evidence that contraceptive counseling and provision has not centered—and does not currently center—the needs, desires, and preferences of women of color. What is notable is that Alexis was eighteen. She formulated her skepticism largely based on knowl-edge of others' experiences and history rather than from her own experience. The result was that Alexis distrusted her doctor, ren-dering any attempt by the physician to allay Alexis's concerns about contraception further evidence of the latter as untrustworthy. At that time, although Alexis did not want to become a parent as a teenager and did not want to have another abortion, her distrust of her doctor and contraception meant that she did not have real access to highly effective, reversible means to prevent another preg-nancy. Alexis was pregnant now because the legacy of medical mistreatment of women of color like those in her community informed her assessment of risks and benefits of using prescrip-tion contraception.

Aside from the specific care they received or did not receive, respondents also articulated an expectation of poor interpersonal treatment from staff and others related to health care. Mariah, from chapter 2, for instance, remarked that she was surprised to be greeted kindly when she first presented for prenatal care, illus-trating the low expectations for care many respondents held. She said: "The lady at the desk was really friendly, which actually hon-estly surprised me because of the area that I'm in. So it really, really surprised me. It was kind of refreshing, especially because of the kind of doctor's office it is accepts Medicaid, and so it's a lot of low-income folks that come in. . . . So the people that work with us low-income folks usually have attitudes, or they're not as friendly or as open or warm or anything like that." Mariah explained that her surprise came from her experience-informed expectation of poor treatment in healthcare settings because of her low-income status. Her past experience of poor treatment is part of a larger pattern of disrespect for low-income patients by healthcare workers (Bridges 2011). In chapter 2, I discussed the structural barriers to abortion Mariah faced. To the extent that her experience of poor treatment by healthcare professionals engendered in her a sense of futility, Mariah may have been unmotivated to continue to try to overcome those structural obstacles to abortion.

These examples illustrate how pregnancy itself alongside decisions about abortion took place in a context characterized by experiences of medical mistreatment and medical mistrust. Scholarship has robustly demonstrated that medical mistrust is the effect—and not the cause—of poor-quality care and medical mistreatment (Boyd et al. 2020). The failure of the healthcare system to equitably serve all populations directly contributed to some respondents' pregnancy circumstances and operated as a constraint on some women's ability to choose abortion. Tying back to anticipated negative embodiment, medical mistrust, in turn, could further foment inequity in reproductive experiences. It meant that respondents did not always see healthcare workers, including abortion providers, as helpers or as people who could address their concerns about the embodied physical and emotional experience of contraception and abortion.

After Anticipated Embodiment

Some of the women whose experiences are recounted in this chapter had adjusted to the idea of having a baby by the time we talked. Madison, for instance, felt good about continuing her pregnancy when we spoke. Others, like Tandra, who hoped for a miscarriage, felt that they could not choose abortion but still hoped the pregnancy would end. And still others, like Deirdre, were nearly distraught about continuing their pregnancy, even as abortion remained unchooseable for them. Deirdre explained to me that she was experiencing deep feelings of sadness and depression unlike any she had ever experienced before—and her family was unsympathetic. She said, "They acting like 'you can't be real' or something. They just don't understand. I've never been at a vulnerable point in my life like this."

Three of the women I interviewed went a different route: they tried to end their pregnancies on their own, outside of the healthcare system. Like the women who made similar attempts discussed in chapter 2, their attempts were unsuccessful. Unlike the women whose accounts were discussed in chapter 2, these three women's attempts to end their pregnancies on their own were informed, at least in part, by their expectations for what the experience of a clinic-supervised abortion would be, rather than in response to structural barriers to clinic-based abortion care. These accounts suggest that abortion outside the healthcare system may be a first choice for some people, rather than a last resort, but also that part of that preference may stem from anticipated negative embodiment of abortion and medical mistrust.

Samantha, a thirty-eight-year-old white woman in Maryland, had expectations of the embodied experience of abortion that were rooted in her prior experience of abortion. Samantha had an abortion as a teenager. Her sexual relationship at the time was coercive: "I don't feel like I always had a say-so in whether we were having sex or not." She did not want to become a parent as a teenager or be tied to this boyfriend, and abortion felt like the right decision. Nonetheless, she experienced her abortion as emotionally difficult. She felt sad about the experience. She said thinking about it "does not feel good to me, like, any of it." In the years since, she has been in healthier relationships and able to manage her fertility, becoming pregnant twice when she wanted to be. More than two decades after her abortion, at thirty-eight, Samantha did not initially recognize her pregnancy symptoms, including not having a period and nausea, attributing them a change in contraceptive method and the stress of a new weight-loss program. Then, one night, she suddenly realized she was pregnant: "I woke up at three o'clock in the morning one day and just knew. I was just like, oh, fuck." She did not want any more children. She told me, "My first reaction was: this is not happening and I wasn't going to keep the baby."

Starting that day and for the next week and a half, she tried to cause an abortion on her own. She took vitamins, drank teas of various herbs, lifted heavy objects, and placed raw parsley in her vagina, all in an effort to end the pregnancy. She knew of abortion clinics. She even had friends who worked at an abortion clinic. But she did not want to go to an abortion clinic. She explained that this was because of her prior experience of abortion: "I didn't necessarily really want to go through with the whole procedure [in a clinic] because I did it when I was fifteen and it sucked. And I felt like it was something that I'd never have to be faced with again. And I was just, you know. The whole thing was super, super sad." Samantha did not regret her prior abortion, but she also did not want to have another abortion—at least not another in-clinic abortion. Ending her pregnancy on her own, for Samantha, was preferable because it would be distinct—and thus not emotionally related—to her abortion at age fifteen. She said, "I just felt like it would have been more private versus something that I had to make a huge ordeal about." In their study of people who sought abortion medications online without clinical supervision, public affairs scholar Abigail Aiken and colleagues (2018) found that, like Samantha, some participants were motivated by a desire for privacy.

Samantha's efforts made her feel sick, but they did not cause an abortion. As Samantha did the math about when she might have conceived, she realized, "I wasn't just brand-new pregnant." The failure of the herbs to end her pregnancy made her realize "I was probably beyond eight weeks if that stuff wasn't working." This changed her thinking about abortion, she explained: "And I'm not, you know—everybody's entitled to their own thing, but having an abortion much later than where I felt like I already was was not even going to be an option for me." Samantha attempted to end her pregnancy on her own out of a desire to avoid associations with her prior experience of abortion. When that failed, her endorsement of a cultural narrative of abortion as killing after fetal personhood is established (for her, around ten weeks into pregnancy) made abortion, with or without clinic supervision, unchooseable. Samantha was continuing her pregnancy.

Sequitta, a thirty-eight-year-old Black woman in Maryland, also tried to end her pregnancy on her own because she wanted to avoid another in-clinic abortion experience. Sequitta had been treated badly by men throughout her life. She said: "That's how the men was in my life. They would call, say they love me, they would abuse me. I used to think that when I got hit on, I used to think that's because they cared about me. Especially the person I was with for ten years, the one I got three kids by, he really used to abuse me. And I'm talking about black eyes, stitches, everything." Her current pregnancy came from a casual relationship with a man she works with. Sequitta wanted another child, but only under specific circumstances. As I described in chapter 1, Sequitta told me, "I do want another child, but I want another child by somebody I'm with and we can raise it together in the same household as a family. Not separate. I feel like I'm just too old for that. Like I just want to settle down, that's all." This man was not going to give her that. Instead, when she told him she was pregnant, she said, "he turned on me and he was just like so mean." She then learned that another co-worker was also pregnant by this man. This did not feel to Sequitta like the right circumstances to have a baby.

At the same time, Sequitta felt like she should not have an abortion because, in her experience of abortion, it could lead to bad outcomes. Specifically, Sequitta attributed a series of bad things that happened to her to one of her prior abortions. She explained: "When I had did that one, it was, like, bad stuff happened. It was like as soon as I came out of the abortion clinic, the police pulled behind me. Took my car because I ain't had no insurance. [Then,] the person that I was pregnant by, he used to take these [pills] and he would be a totally different person. And he almost killed me that night. So he, yes, he tried to throw me off a third-floor building. I just felt like, oh, that was bad luck for what I had done." Sequitta believed that her abortion caused the violence she experienced and the bad luck of being caught without proof of insurance by the police. The mechanism through which that would happen is difficult to imagine. And she had no such problems after her other abortions. Here, however, I am not interested in the empirical veracity of her logic but rather in the way her embodied experience of abortion elastically includes non-health-related outcomes—and negative ones, at that.

Even as she did not wish to have another baby, Sequitta felt constrained by what choosing abortion meant. She hoped to cause a miscarriage by drinking wine: "Instead of me getting the abortion [at a clinic], I was trying to drink a lot." She drank at least a bottle each time, more frequently soon after discovering the pregnancy and less frequently by the time of the interview, in the middle of her second trimester. It did not cause a miscarriage. Still, in her independent efforts to end her pregnancy, Sequitta avoided experiential association with an in-clinic abortion. During this time, she scheduled and failed to show up for multiple abortion appointments, each time oscillating between a desire not to be pregnant and feeling unable to experience another clinic-based abortion. If the pregnancy ended because of her drinking, she reasoned, that was not the same as having another abortion—and would not carry the same risk of consequences. The alcohol also helped her navigate the loneliness and isolation she felt, facing another pregnancy with a man who did not care for her.

The last respondent who attempted to end her pregnancy on her own because of, in part, anticipated negative embodiment of abortion was Sonja. Unlike Samantha and Sequitta, Sonja, a twenty-six-year-old Black woman in Louisiana, had never had an abortion. Nonetheless, as she learned about what an in-clinic abortion would entail, she was fearful of the embodied experience of having one. Sonja was homeless, and she and one of her daughters were sleeping on a cousin's couch. As I mentioned in chapter 1, her older daughter was living with another family member in a functional synergy because Sonja could not provide her with a stable environment and the family member needed additional help at home. Another relative had recently been murdered, and Sonja was working through deep emotional trauma following his death. Seeking comfort, Sonja had a casual sexual relationship with a man who was already in a relationship with someone else. His existing commitment had initially made Sonja feel better about being with him: he could not expect a commitment from her, and she was uninterested in making one. Sonja hoped to have another child someday, but it was not the right time, and this was not the right man. As she summarized, "I'm not in my own house or anything and I was going through a lot of stuff at the time when I did find out. And I was like oh, I just felt like I couldn't bring no child into the world."

When Sonja realized she was pregnant, she first thought, "I really wasn't going to keep the baby." She had been raised to understand abortion as morally wrong, however, so considering abortion was complicated for her. When she sought input from the man involved, this complexity increased. He pressured her to continue the pregnancy, wanting to be connected to her long term. This was unpersuasive to her. As she explained, "I didn't want to deal with him, but he wanted to deal with me. . . . I don't want to be in no relationship with him. He wants a relationship and I don't want no relationship with him." He expressed strong opposition to abortion.

After telling the man involved, Sonja kept the pregnancy to herself, focusing on her own mental health, trying to create a stable life for her daughters, and ignoring the pregnancy. When I asked what was happening in her life at that time and why she waited to call a clinic, she said, "I don't know. I really can't tell you. I don't know why. You said why? I don't know." She was grappling with her personal opposition to abortion, but explained that was not the whole reason for her delay in calling: "I really don't believe in it [abortion], but it was something I was going to do, like

I said, because at the time, like I told you, I was going through stuff in my life."

Two months after discovering her pregnancy, she called an abortion clinic and learned of all the things she would have to undergo during the appointment: "You have to watch some videos to make sure you could go through the procedure, but you still have the right to change your mind. After you see the video, you have the right to change your mind if you want to do that or not." Sonja found it difficult to imagine watching the video and then proceeding to abortion. Like Mercedes, she felt certain that she would decline to have an abortion if subjected to this anticipated in-clinic experience. In this way, a structural obstacle to abortion featured in her abortion decision making. Its mechanism for doing so, however, was by complicating her anticipated embodiment of abortion. It informed how she imagined the experience of getting an abortion.

Even as Sonja ruled out going to an abortion clinic, she still wanted to end her pregnancy. At around five months pregnant, she took both prescription and recreational drugs in an attempt to cause a miscarriage. Neither drug is an abortifacient, but Sonja still hoped they would end her pregnancy "because it was drugs. I feel like if you take so many of them, it'll do something." While she could not imagine getting an abortion at a clinic and experiencing the state-mandated counseling, she could imagine ending her own pregnancy. She said, "If it had worked at the time that I wanted it to, I probably would have been happy." As it was, "it didn't do nothing."

Conclusion

The anticipated embodied experience of abortion, including anticipation based on past experience of abortion and of health care can influence current pregnancy decision making. In this chapter, I have shown how some respondents anticipated that the embodied experience of abortion would be negative, and this constrained their ability to choose abortion after considering it. For some, the rhetorical availability of abortion to be causal meant that they associated negative feelings and experiences with abortion itself, assigning blame to abortion rather than to the circumstances in which the abortion took place. When abortion itself was understood as causal—and as causing bad things—respondents imagined that having an abortion would lead to bad outcomes. This could make it unchooseable. For others, the dearth of providers meant that they were unable to secure the conditions of care they sought for abortion. They wanted to terminate their pregnancy, but they had expectations of the circumstances under which they would obtain an abortion. Absent those conditions of care, abortion was unchooseable. For all these respondents, their anticipated experiences of abortion, importantly, were rooted in the body, in what they imagined the embodied experience of abortion would be.

In parallel to these anticipated bodily experiences, respondents evidenced mistrust of healthcare workers. Several offered examples of specific medical mistreatment that engendered their distrust, including healthcare failures that contributed to them being pregnant. Their anticipated negative embodied experience of abortion, then, should be understood as about more than the specifics of abortion. Their concerns about what an embodied experience of abortion would be are, yes, tied to antiabortion cultural narratives and informed by structural barriers to abortion. They are also effects of the failures of healthcare systems to equitably care for all patients. Abortion can become unchooseable because the healthcare system has not earned the trust of women like these respondents.

6

Choosing a Baby

For the women whose accounts I have shared in the previous chapters, as I have shown, there was no real pregnancy decision. In various ways, including structural barriers, antiabortion cultural narratives, and anticipated negative embodiment, abortion was unchooseable for them, and thus pregnancies were continued, whether the respondent eventually wanted to have a baby or not. There was one group of respondents, however, whose continuation of pregnancy is not explained by the abortion as unchooseable framework. A small number of respondents who considered but did not obtain an abortion did so for a very simple reason: they wanted to have a baby.

Shakeia, a twenty-four-year-old Black woman in Louisiana, for example, wanted to continue her pregnancy and have a third child but was uncertain if these were the right circumstances. She wanted her existing and future children to have a father figure, and she wanted someone who would share parenting responsibilities with her. She and her boyfriend of five months were discussing whether they wanted to stay together around the time she discovered she was pregnant. The father of her five-year-old and two-year-old did not participate in their lives, and Shakeia feared that "with this one I was going to be stuck in the same boat. I wasn't going to have help like I wanted it." She considered abortion—and she constructed this consideration as normal. She said, "I mean, at first every woman has that thought of, should I abort? Should I keep it? What should I do? The only way they're not going to have that thought is if they're in a very good, successful relationship at the time, meaning that they have no financial problems or anything like that." She wanted to continue this pregnancy, but only if her boyfriend would be an involved father.

When she told him about the pregnancy, her worries about being a single parent to another child were assuaged. She said:

> I told him, and I was just like I was scared, not only scared, but I was just worried about me having another child and being a single mother with three kids and trying to make it on my own. And that's when he said to me, "You don't have to worry about that." He was like, "You don't have to worry about that with me. I'm going to be there with you, all the way, you know. This is my first child. I'm just as excited as you are. And I want to see you go through everything in a positive way, not in a negative way." So, he was like, I got your back.

Shakeia felt immense relief. Her concerns about continuing this pregnancy were mitigated. The circumstances for having this baby were the circumstances she wanted. She was no longer interested in abortion. She wanted to have a baby. In this chapter, I examine the experiences of respondents like Shakeia who continued their pregnancies because they wanted a baby.

In tracing the experiences of the women featured in this chapter, I elucidate an intriguing discursive practice: their detailed accounts did not always align with their summary explanations of what was consequential to their pregnancy decision. Specifically, when they summarized their pregnancy decision making, they did not always include their desire for a baby. Instead, their simplified explanations tended to feature reasons why they could not and would not choose abortion and to deploy antiabortion cultural narratives. Shakeia is again an example. While Shakeia presented consideration of abortion as normal at the outset of our interview, that frame shifted as we talked. Recounting conversations with others about abortion later in our interview, Shakeia endorsed the idea of abortion as killing, expressing sadness and guilt that she had ever considered abortion. She said, "It made me real sad because I'm like, wow, that makes me a murderer. Even I thought about it, so that makes me a murderer just because I thought about it." She avowed that she would never choose abortion because it is murder. In so doing, she invoked an antiabortion cultural narrative to explain her pregnancy outcome, even as, by her own account, it was not a factor during her decision making. While the cultural narrative of abortion as killing was not what motivated her to continue her pregnancy—her desire for a baby and her boyfriend's investment in the pregnancy were what mattered for her decision making—Shakeia utilized it to make sense of that consideration after the fact.

This use follows sociologist Ann Swidler's (2001) generative concept of cultural repertoires wherein one justifies or explains an action by deploying particular cultural accounts, or repertoires. As I will show was the case for the respondents discussed in this chapter, people can use accounts to explain or justify an action that does not match up with the behavior that preceded or compelled the action. Some of this is about what is discursively available. At any time, people have a finite set of accounts and representations available to them. But I suggest that, for these respondents, perhaps unconsciously, these cultural deployments also had a benefit: they enabled respondents to frame their continuation of pregnancy in a socially accepted way—that is, as a rejection of abortion. As I explicate below, childbearing by low-income women and women of color has been broadly maligned. There are, accordingly, few social narratives of choosing to have a baby available to pregnant women such as the women I interviewed, most of whom were poor and Black. By framing their continuation of pregnancy as about not choosing abortion—rather than as about choosing to have a baby—respondents could discursively bypass social judgment of their decision to parent under circumstances that do not match raced and classed normative ideals. This use underscores not only the dominance of antiabortion cultural narratives for making sense of pregnancy decision making but also the absence of cultural narratives affirming low-income women's and women of color's right to parent.

Wanting a Baby

Representing a small number of the women I interviewed, ten respondents considered but did not obtain an abortion because they wanted a baby. Of these, a handful reported that they initially thought about abortion because they worried that they could not safely continue their pregnancy because of health reasons. In Renita's case, it was her own health that was of concern. About a year ago, Renita, a thirty-eight-year-old Black woman in Louisiana, was hospitalized with a serious medical condition. Her doctors were able to stabilize her, but she continued to take several medications to manage her condition. Her pregnancy was a surprise. At thirty-eight, Renita had been pregnant only once before, and the pregnancy ended in miscarriage. Even as her friends had babies, Renita had not. She had come to terms with the idea that she might never become a mother. As she said, "I'm not one of those people who kept trying, kept trying, but there was times when, yeah, I wanted to [become a mother]." This felt like her chance. When she learned she was pregnant, she said, "I was happy." Her pre-existing medical condition, however, complicated her pregnancy. Her doctors worried that continuing the pregnancy would exacerbate her condition. It had been barely a year since her initial hospitalization, and her condition was not stable. They also communicated concerns about the effects of the medications she took on fetal development. The medications are not recommended for pregnancy, but her doctors also assessed that it was imperative to her health that she continue to take them. As Renita related, "the benefits outweigh the risks." Ultimately, given her current health, her doctors recommended she terminate the pregnancy. Her family agreed, insisting that she prioritize her health.

Renita recognized the risk she was taking in being pregnant and thought about abortion. Her body felt bad, making her worry that her condition was worsening. She explained, "I was thinking, if I'm going to be sick like this, I don't know if I can do it, physically if my body would do it." Notably, in contrast to the women in earlier chapters, Renita felt able to choose abortion. Her family supported her choosing abortion. And her physicians not only supported her choosing abortion, they went so far as to offer to facilitate an abortion at the hospital because of her health conditions, enabling her to use insurance coverage and eliminating any funding concerns. But Renita wanted a baby. She sought and received emotional support for continuing the pregnancy at an antiabortion pregnancy resource center (see also Kimport 2019, 2020). She feared missing the opportunity to have a baby more than the health risks of continuing the pregnancy. She fastened onto the possibility that there could be no health problems in continuing the pregnancy: "What if they were wrong? What if I was to deliver it healthy? What if everything would've went okay? I don't want to go through the rest of my life thinking that." In deciding between abortion and continuing the pregnancy, Renita decided to continue her pregnancy. She told me, "No matter what I'm going to continue with it."

In her pregnancy, Sabrina, a thirty-two-year-old Black woman in Louisiana, was not worried about her own health, but feared that her opioid use would negatively affect fetal development. When Sabrina discovered she was pregnant, she was happy. She was using a long-acting contraceptive method, so was initially "shocked" to be pregnant, but she was also excited to have a baby. This was tempered with her understanding that using opioids during pregnancy was not a good idea. She explained, "I was extremely happy and excited that I'm having a baby, but, you know, that's it. I was just happy I was having my baby, but I couldn't be happy because I was so worried and stressed out because I knew what I was doing [using opioids], you know?" She and her partner of eleven years discussed abortion because they believed her use of opioids during pregnancy would harm the fetus. While research does find short-term harms of maternal opioid use, such as neonatal opioid withdrawal syndrome, it has not documented any long-term adverse impacts of opioid use during pregnancy (Conradt et al. 2019). As Sabrina considered abortion as a possibility, she weighed it against her desire to continue the pregnancy. She said, "That [abortion] was something that I thought about. But I just didn't go through with it because I wanted my baby. I didn't want to terminate it." As Sabrina concisely stated, she continued her pregnancy because she wanted a baby. After trying two different obstetricians, she finally found a doctor who could help her safely manage her opioid use during pregnancy.

Other respondents who continued their pregnancies because they wanted a baby considered abortion only at the prompting of others in their lives. Jade, a twenty-nine-year-old Black woman in Louisiana, was one example. Jade's family had recently experienced a trauma, and she was unsure whether she, her fiancé, and her two daughters had the energy, resources, and support to, as she described it, "start over" with a new baby. When she told her fiancé and children about the pregnancy, though, they were excited, seeing the pregnancy as an opportunity for change and love after an especially difficult time for their family. For Jade, a new baby was something to look forward to. She told me, "I'm just ready to get my life started back right."

Jade told two friends about her pregnancy in passing, and they reacted differently. As Jade recounted, "They were sort of negative just about me wanting to have another baby and starting all over and saying what all I would end up going through and this and that or whatever." They encouraged her to consider abortion "before it gets too late." Jade was not especially close to these two friends, but she thought about what they said for a day or so. She felt, she said, "confused." She was excited about a baby, but also aware that she and her family were still recovering from a trauma. Maybe, she thought, this was not the right time to have a baby. Her friends' comments made her think, but they did not make her feel pressured. In contrast to the experiences of coercion referenced in chapter 5, Jade experienced this abortion suggestion as simply a suggestion. As she mulled it over, she felt clarity that she wanted a baby. In the end, she felt like she had made an active choice to continue her pregnancy. She related, "I'm kind of glad I thought about it . . . because I can distinguish the difference now."

Gabriella's consideration of abortion was also brief and prompted by a conversation. Gabriella, a twenty-eight-year-old Black woman in Maryland, and her husband were planning to move and feeling some financial strain around this plan. They needed more space for their two existing children, but worried about affording rent on a bigger home. When Gabriella missed her period, she knew she was pregnant. She felt happy. She and her husband had talked about having another child. She told her husband she thought she was pregnant, and he asked her "do I want to keep it? Are we ready for another baby? Like stuff like that." They discussed it together, deciding that they both wanted a baby and could manage their financial struggles. It felt to Gabriella like a reasonable conversation to have, and she was satisfied with the outcome.

Finally, like Shakeia from the opening of the chapter, a few respondents who wanted to have a baby explained that they considered abortion because, initially, they were unsure their circumstances were right for having a baby. Once they felt confident the circumstances were good, or good enough, to parent in—in Shakeia's case, once she got a commitment of support from her boyfriend—they chose to continue their pregnancies.

Each of these respondents continued her pregnancy because she wanted a baby. It sounds simple. But, as earlier chapters illustrated, that was not the case for most of the women I interviewed. While some of the women whose accounts were discussed in earlier chapters came to desire a baby—and many did not—the consequential reason they were continuing their pregnancies was that they were unable to choose abortion. That was not so for the women in this chapter.

Explaining Their Decision

Yet, when most of these women explained why they were continuing their pregnancies, they deployed at least one of the antiabortion cultural narratives described in chapters 3 and 4, rather than citing their desire to have a baby. This pattern highlights not only the ubiquity of antiabortion cultural narratives but also the dearth of cultural narratives affirming low-income and poor Black women's right to parent. Patrice, a twenty-seven-year-old Black woman in Maryland, is one example. Patrice had her first child when she was a young teenager. She tried to care for him for his first four months but was unsuccessful. Unable to raise him, she granted a close family friend custody to raise him as her own son. Her current pregnancy, more than a decade later, was a surprise, but a happy surprise. Patrice was eager to become a parent and raise a child. As she told me, "I wanted the chance to have another baby." Ongoing health issues, however, dampened her excitement about the pregnancy. She had diagnosed clinical depression, anxiety, and insomnia. About a year prior, Patrice began having unexplained seizures. She had seen multiple doctors and tried multiple medications. However, not only did the seizures persist, but no doctor had been able to diagnose the cause. Patrice was worried about the effect of the various medications, including antidepressants, sleep aids, and anti-seizure medications, on fetal development and what would happen if, despite those medications, she continued to have seizures. She explained: "I mean, I was kind of happy [to be pregnant], but it was just like, at the same time, I was afraid for the baby, because I knew my current health status with the seizures, and I know what happens when I have them. I fall, I bust up, I got stitches, my tongue is split, like I don't want to be pregnant and have to have the baby go through that. I don't know what will happen." Patrice, in other words, wanted to have a baby—"I actually want it," she said—but, like Renita and Sabrina, was concerned about the health risk.

Researching the effects of her medications on pregnancy on the Internet did not help. She reported: "I was just looking up a bunch of stuff, and it scared me. . . . There was stuff saying I could die, and the baby could die. . . . I'm not trying to die. I'm trying to live. I don't want to bring this baby in this world and die." She thought about abortion as a possibility. In her thinking, though, abortion was "just a back-up thing. . . . And if they [my doctors] tell me something bad [about my condition or medication] or they tell me,

'What I'm seeing on the computer [is bad],' then that would just be an option." Once her obstetrician told her it was okay for her to continue to use most of her medications and switched one that was not recommended for use during pregnancy, she said, "I was feeling a little better." It put her "at ease" with continuing the pregnancy.

When she summed up her abortion consideration later in our interview, however, she added a component. Citing the abortion as harmful cultural narrative that constructs abortion as causing mental health harms (see chapter 4), Patrice told me that, after considering abortion, she decided, "I'm not going to do that, because I don't want to be depressed all over again." Patrice had not had a prior abortion. Her reference to being depressed "all over again" was in regard to her history of depression, not personal abortion experience. This explanation for why she was continuing her pregnancy did not accord with her account of the salient aspects of her decision making when she walked me step by step through her pregnancy experience to date. Most specifically, this explanation did not highlight her desire for a baby. It was, nonetheless, expedient in her short version of why she was continuing her pregnancy. It also deflected attention from potential challenges to the suitability of her continuing a pregnancy. By accounting for her pregnancy decision making through recourse to cultural narratives about why she should not choose abortion, Patrice did not have to defend her choice to have a baby.

Destiny, a twenty-one-year-old Black woman in Maryland, employed a similar discursive strategy. When Destiny learned she was pregnant, she and her boyfriend of nine months were excited about having a baby. She told me, "I was happy . . . that I got blessed to be able to be healthy enough to carry a child." Leading up to the pregnancy, she said, there were times when she wanted to become pregnant—and times when she did not. When she discovered she was pregnant, it felt right to have a baby. Her aunt disagreed. As Destiny described, "She sent me a text message saying that I'm not going to be able to take care of the baby 'cause I'm not able to take care of myself." Other family members were doubtful of Destiny and her boyfriend's ability to be responsible for a baby, too, and they admonished that "it's time to be serious," getting jobs and moving out of her boyfriend's family's house to their own place. Destiny's aunt implied that a different route was better: ending the pregnancy.

Destiny was offended at her aunt's suggestion that she was unprepared to become a parent and angry at her aunt for suggesting abortion. She said, "It made me really upset." When Destiny was unhappy with her boyfriend, however, she thought about what her aunt said. She explained that she considered abortion "when my baby's father smokes his cigarettes, like around me. Like not close to me but around me, and I tell him to go somewhere else because the smell start making me feel nauseous." She elaborated, "I would feel physically bad, and then mentally angry at him. And I would start getting all these extreme emotions, so that [abortion] would come into my head. But then once I calmed down, it goes away." Destiny's consideration of abortion was sparked by her aunt's comment, but her interest in choosing abortion never progressed beyond those few moments of intense anger. She said of abortion, "I'm not really interested in it." She wanted to have a baby.

Later in the interview, however, when she accounted for why she decided to continue her pregnancy, she drew on the cultural narrative of abortion as against God's will. She told me she would never obtain an abortion because "I kind of like don't really think it's right in the eyes of God. . . . I just feel like it's morally wrong." This antiabortion cultural narrative, in other words, took on explanatory power for her actions after the fact. This phenomenon of drawing on an existing cultural narrative to explain or justify an action is an exemplar of Swidler's (2001) idea of cultural repertoires. These narratives served as a shorthand for making sense of these women's actions, even as respondents' statements and their reported actions were not always in alignment.

Neither Patrice nor Destiny described their deployment of antiabortion cultural narratives as strategic. But there are reasons to consider this discursive framing of their pregnancy decision making as such. Scholars have shown that policy and media coverage often constructs women in their social location—low-income and/ or poor mothers of color—as a drain on public resources (Benson-smith 2005; D. Roberts 1999; Thomas 1998). Research shows how policies as well as providers of reproductive health care treat these women's desire to reproduce with suspicion (Downing, LaVeist, and Bullock 2007), constructing it as a nefarious ploy to reap more money from public sources (B. Wilcox et al. 1996) or as stemming from ignorance as to their inadequacy as a potential parent (Stevens 2015). Ideals of "appropriate motherhood" are both raced and classed, premised on a middle-class white woman as the norm (Collins 2006; Stevens 2015; Thomas 1998). As anthropologists Faye Ginsburg and Rayna Rapp (1995) cogently argued, reproduction is stratified, with greater social value accorded to procreation by white and more affluent women than to procreation by low-income and poor women and women of color. Women like these respondents, whose procreation is not socially valued, are then called upon to justify their desire to reproduce (Killen 2019; Luna and Luker 2013; Ross and Solinger 2017). By framing their continuation of pregnancy as a rejection of abortion, however, Patrice and Destiny avoid that discursive terrain. They rhetorically deploy a different set of cultural narratives about pregnancy—that is, antiabortion narratives—that position their continuation of pregnancy favor-ably. Narratives that reframe pregnancy decision making as about whether to choose abortion, in other words, can enable women whose right to parent is doubted to explain their decision in socially rewarded terms.

Role of Important Others

The social components of this framing are evident in Abigail's account. Her after-the-fact repertoire deployment was aided by language from others. Abigail, a thirty-two-year-old white woman in Maryland, thought seriously about abortion when she discov-ered her pregnancy for several reasons. Her controlling and vio-lent ex-boyfriend had prevented her from seeing her two children (ages seven and five) for the last few years, even though they lived nearby. This devastated her. She felt she had little recourse, however, since she had a history of opioid use and had only been clean for a year. When she first left him, she explained, "his family stepped in because they have money, and they threatened me if I went to court that they had money, they'd win, and that they would hurt me and all this old crazy stuff." After the hostility she faced from her ex and his family in the past, she feared that any new dynamic in their relationship, such as having a new baby, would impede her ability to reconnect with her existing children.

There was another dimension to her fear. Abigail is white, and her boyfriend of four years is Black. Although white women's right to parent has not been systematically questioned the way women of color's right to parent has (Collins 2006; Luna and Luker 2013; D. Roberts 1999; Ross and Solinger 2017), Abigail was aware of how race mattered in her situation. Her ex is white and racist. When she was still in contact with him about their shared children, he made clear his disapproval of her current boyfriend because he is Black through an aggressive display along with numerous racist comments. Abigail knew that having a child with her Black boyfriend would enrage her ex and believed it would make him more adamant that she could not see her existing children.

Separate from her fears related to her relationships with her existing children, Abigail was also scared about whether, being so newly clean, she was ready for a new baby. She worried about the small apartment she and her boyfriend lived in and the fact that she did not have a job. Abortion, in some moments, meant she could be closer to her ideal circumstances for parenting, having more space and financial stability.

Abigail also wanted a baby. She felt like having a baby "gives me another chance to be a mom again." And unlike in her previous relationship, she had the support she wanted from her caring boyfriend. He told her, she related, "'I'll be there 100 percent. I love you.'" After her violent and inconsistent ex, Abigail finally felt safe and supported with her current boyfriend.

Caught between a desire for a baby and fear of permanent loss of her relationships with her existing children, Abigail made an appointment for an abortion without telling her boyfriend. When they called her name at the appointment, she got up and walked out. She decided that, with her boyfriend's support, these were good enough circumstances for having a baby and that she would risk the effect on her access to her existing children. She could face her fears of becoming a mother again. When she told her boyfriend about having gone to the abortion clinic, he both deferred to her right to make a pregnancy decision and invoked a narrative of abortion as killing. As Abigail recounted, "He was like, 'If that's what you would've wanted, I wouldn't have stopped you.' He was like, 'But think about it, that's a human being.' I was like, 'Yeah, you're right.'" In Abigail's account, she decided not to obtain an abortion and then, after discussing her actions with her boyfriend, was presented with and agreed with the cultural narrative that abortion is killing.

This narrative of abortion as killing then dominated her summarization of her experience. Abigail told me she decided against abortion because "I was just like, just couldn't kill it. That's all I kept thinking was, like, [it] didn't ask to be here." In this concise explanation of her pregnancy outcome, Abigail did not reference her fears about staying clean, that continuing the pregnancy would render her estrangement from her existing children permanent, or about having adequate space for a baby. These are more personal factors and specific to her life circumstances. Nor did she state that she engaged with those fears and weighed them against her desire for a baby, deciding that she could be a successful parent under her current conditions. Instead, her simple explanation deployed the antiabortion cultural narrative that abortion is killing. I do not mean to suggest that Abigail did not hold this belief, or that it was simply convenient for her to deploy this cultural narrative. Instead, what Abigail's account illustrates is the way that antiabortion cultural narratives are available and, in Abigail's case, a useful shorthand for justifying one's pregnancy outcome. To the extent that cultural narratives are structured as common sense, it also enabled Abigail to avoid having to justify continuation of a pregnancy she was still unsure she could financially support and for which she did not feel she embodied ideal parenting circumstances—and a pregnancy that, because of her racist ex's actions, could mean loss of her motherhood role for her other children. Though she did not reference how being relatively newly clean mattered, deploying antiabortion cultural narratives may also have enabled her to avoid social suspicion of pregnant and parenting women who use or have used drugs (Flavin 2008; Flavin and Paltrow 2010). In other words, rather than having to defend her desire to parent—and recalling that others had questioned her right to parent in the past—Abigail opted to cite a justification for continuing her pregnancy that positioned her as a good, moral person.

Conclusion

As these cases illustrate, some of the women I interviewed considered and did not obtain an abortion because they wanted to have a baby. Their experiences conformed more closely to the broad social narrative of pregnancy decision making: they chose between having an abortion and continuing their pregnancy. They were not, like the women from previous chapters, continuing their pregnancies because abortion was unchooseable. Antiabortion cultural narratives nonetheless shadow many of their accounts. These narratives were used to justify, after the fact, some respondents' decisions not to obtain an abortion. They served as a useful shorthand for explaining their pregnancy outcomes, even as they did not accurately capture respondents' step-by-step accounts of their decision making.

Deploying antiabortion cultural narratives to retroactively explain continuation of pregnancy was expedient for these women. It helped sum up an outcome using normatively accepted language and deflected attention from the ways, both within and beyond their control, they did not embody society's racist and classed normative ideals for motherhood. In this way, I demonstrate that antiabortion cultural narratives do not solely motivate action in women's pregnancy decision making, as I described in chapters 3 and 4. They also can be used to explain decisions in socially acceptable logics. In this second way, these narratives become hegemonic, dominating and limiting discursive opportunities for making sense of pregnancy decision making. Their use by respondents who continued their pregnancies expressly because they wanted a baby reveals the parallel absence of cultural narratives available to low-income women and women of color to explain and justify their desire to parent.

7
Toward Reproductive Autonomy

Not everyone who continues a pregnancy wants a baby. Sometimes, people are doing so because they cannot afford an abortion; because they cannot find a provider; because they do not trust the provider they can find; because the narratives available to them construct abortion as killing, against God's will, irresponsible, or causing them harm; because a previous experience made them promise never to have another abortion. These are ways abortion becomes unchooseable, even when it is legal and ostensibly available. These are not reasons for having a baby.

The normative narrative of pregnancy decision making as a choice between continuation and termination, however, has no space for these experiences. Instead, it is premised on an assumption I have shown to be faulty: that pregnant people are able to choose between abortion and continuation. This assumption is so widely held as to preclude our ability to discuss it. When public, policy, and private discussions assume pregnant women have a real choice in their pregnancy outcome, the pregnancy decision making of most of the women I interviewed is misunderstood and the constraints on their reproductive autonomy reified.

This is an injustice. Some readers will focus specifically on the fact that so many of the women I interviewed were prevented from obtaining an abortion, considering barriers to abortion of greatest concern. But the injustice I am interested in precedes respondents' pregnancy outcomes. The injustice I am interested in here is that these women had no true pregnancy choice. When abortion was unchooseable, they could not engage in pregnancy decision making that centered their wants, their circumstances, and the input of important others. When abortion was unchooseable, their decision-making process was not about clarifying their pregnancy desires or resolving ambivalence about choosing between abortion and having a baby. Indeed, in a scenario where abortion were chooseable, some respondents might have chosen to continue their pregnancy, illustrating that pregnancy outcome alone is not evidence of reproductive autonomy or lack thereof. Instead, however, these women's pregnancy decision making was curtailed by structural and cultural constraints on their reproductive agency and autonomy, impeding not just their ability to choose abortion but also their ability to choose the circumstances under which they wanted to parent. This injustice is about reproductive agency and autonomy in making a pregnancy decision.

Further, in concert with the absence of cultural narratives that affirm the right of low-income and poor women and women of color to parent, the injustice of unchooseable abortion extended to respondents who continued their pregnancies because they wanted to have a baby. The hegemony of abortion as unchooseable meant that many in this subset deployed accounts of pregnancy decision making that did not center their wants, their circumstances, and the input of important others but, rather, featured a claim that abortion, writ large, is unchooseable. This is a case of utilizing available cultural narratives to explain and justify action (Swidler 2001). That these women's desire and right to parent were not centered in their own storytelling points to the failure of the extant cultural repertoire of narratives as well as a perhaps unexpected consequence of the dominance of antiabortion cultural narratives: constraints on some women's storytelling about their desire to have a baby.

In this concluding chapter, I summarize how and for whom abortion can become unchooseable, denying real choice in pregnancy. The production of abortion as unchooseable I describe is largely specific to the experiences of pregnant people in socially marginalized groups, representing a process that depends on existing race and class inequality. Then, I turn to a discussion of the origins and perpetuation of constraints on choosing abortion. I argue that the antiabortion movement has been more successful than often recognized in making abortion unchooseable. While scholarly attention has been paid to its role in imposing structural barriers to abortion (Hull and Hoffer 2010) and generating antiabortion cultural narratives (Ehrlich and Doan 2019; Kelly 2014; Ludlow 2008; Taylor 1992), my analysis reveals the myriad on-the-ground impacts of antiabortion efforts on individual pregnant women's ability to choose abortion. Still, the antiabortion movement is neither the sole nor the singular force constraining pregnant people's reproductive autonomy, with poverty and medical racism additional contributors. Finally, I close with consideration of what true reproductive autonomy would look like for the women I interviewed.

The Abortion as Unchooseable Framework

Drawing on the experiences of the women I interviewed, I have argued for the utility of an abortion as unchooseable framework. I demonstrated that pregnant women may consider but not obtain an abortion because abortion is unchooseable, not because they want to have a baby—and that abortion became unchooseable for these women, in part, because of race, class, and gender inequality. With abortion unchooseable, they have no real choice.

One way abortion became unchooseable for respondents was through structures. My findings build on research showing that restrictions, especially the ban on public insurance coverage of abortion (Cook et al. 1999; S. Roberts, Johns, et al. 2019), prevent pregnant people from obtaining abortions. When they did not have the money to pay for abortion, for example, they could not choose abortion. The marginalization of abortion care from mainstream medicine, too, made abortion unchooseable for some by making abortion care hard or impossible to find. Abortion was unchooseable for some respondents because they could not find an abortion provider who would care for them.

How these structural obstacles made abortion unchooseable owed to respondents' marginalized social location. The women I interviewed were low income or poor, and most identified as Black. Many of the structural obstacles to abortion that they faced were consequential because of their social location, including policies not formally related to abortion that either perpetuated class inequality or failed to account for a differential impact on people in poverty. Although more of the respondents in Louisiana described what I identify as structural barriers to choosing abortion, abortion was unchooseable because of structural barriers for several Maryland respondents as well. Taken together, their experiences reveal that, while policies restricting abortion are consequential to some women's ability to choose abortion, the underlying condition that renders many of them able to be consequential is poverty—and poverty is not exclusive to states, like Louisiana, with a large number of restrictions on abortion. Pregnant people facing economic insecurity are not only more likely to consider abortion than those who are financially secure, they are also more likely to experience structural barriers to abortion (S. Roberts, Berglas, and Kimport 2020). My analysis illustrates why: poverty makes some barriers to abortion insurmountable. Because poverty is linked to race and both historical and contemporary structural racism in the United States (Baradaran 2017; Branch and Jackson 2020; Oliver and Shapiro 2006), respondents' racial identity mattered for how structural barriers made abortion unchooseable, too.

Importantly, structural barriers could make abortion unchooseable prior to respondents ever contacting an abortion provider, because they intersected with hostility to abortion from loved ones, and/or because respondents lacked trusted resources to fact check misinformation about abortion. Moreover, it bears underscoring that respondents' accounts illustrate how structural barriers to abortion do not operate: they do not prevent abortion by causing women to desire to have a baby; rather, by leveraging existing social inequalities, they make abortion unchooseable, constructing insurmountable barriers to abortion. By utilizing an abortion as unchooseable framework, the structural barriers constraining people's ability to choose abortion, when they curtail decision making, and how class and race matter for that constraint are brought into relief.

Structural barriers were not the only factor that made abortion unchooseable for respondents and impeded their reproductive autonomy. Cultural narratives of what choosing abortion means, serving as internalized and even unconscious ways of understanding the world (Vaisey 2009), made abortion unchooseable for some women. Respondents who understood abortion as killing or as against their god's will found abortion unchooseable. Their understandings of what abortion means in relation to the fetus meant that abortion could not be chosen. To do so, they felt, would be to negate their religious identity and/or their sense of themselves as moral actors. Similarly, respondents who subscribed to cultural narratives of abortion as sexually irresponsible or as causing them physical, mental, and/or emotional harms determined they could not choose abortion. Under these beliefs, choosing abortion meant negating their self-identity as responsible people and/or causing themselves future harm. These meanings for abortion were ubiquitous. Many respondents had no alternative ways of making sense of choosing abortion. Ultimately, the meanings of abortion these narratives presented—alongside the absence of resonant alternative narratives—could make abortion unchooseable.

Without attention to how the power and prevalence of anti-abortion cultural narratives made abortion unchooseable, these women's pregnancy outcomes might be understood as expressions of their personal preference: that they simply wanted to continue their pregnancies. Such an understanding, however, fails to recognize the extent to which antiabortion framing has infiltrated individual women's pregnancy decision making such that they had no real choice, and how patterns of class inequality and racism make some women more at risk of that infiltration. To the extent that consideration of abortion is more common among people who are pregnant when they do not want to be, disparities in family planning (Dehlendorf et al. 2010), many of which are rooted in racism, contribute to low-income and poor women of color being especially likely to be in a situation where they would consider abortion and thus subject to antiabortion cultural narratives. With an abortion as unchooseable framework, their continuation of pregnancy is legible as a response to being unable to choose abortion. Rather than representing a choice that reflects their wants and desires, this continuation is an effect of their lack of reproductive agency.

Finally, respondents' embodied experiences of health care, including abortion, could make abortion unchooseable. Negative experiences of the circumstances around a prior abortion, especially when respondents understood the abortion itself to have caused their negative experience, could make abortion unchooseable. When respondents drew on experience-informed belief that abortion caused them emotional difficulty or physical harm, they anticipated that the embodied experience of a future abortion would be similarly negative, and that made abortion unchooseable for this pregnancy. This process reveals how abortion has been rhetorically constructed as a causal event. Likewise, their expectations for the conditions of abortion care and predictions that undesired conditions would lead to a negative embodied experience of abortion could make abortion unchooseable. Respondents did not simply want an abortion; they wanted an abortion under certain conditions. Absent those conditions of care, abortion was not chooseable. In addition to the specifics of abortion care mattering for many respondents, some described experiences and knowledge of medical racism and mistreatment of vulnerable populations. Obstetric mistreatment could make subsequent abortion more complicated and/or reduce their trust in healthcare workers, removing one potential resource for navigating other structural and cultural barriers to abortion. Such experiences of medical mistrust, engendered by a history of racist medical mistreatment, are higher among people of color than white people (LaVeist, Rolley, and Diala 2003). Its role in making abortion unchooseable for several respondents is therefore particular to the social experience of being a Black woman in the United States.

Women for whom medical experiences and anticipated embodiment of abortion rendered abortion unchooseable are ill-captured by the normative narrative of pregnancy decision making as a real choice. Applying an abortion as unchooseable framework, however, highlights the importance of anticipated embodiment of abortion, the rhetorical availability of abortion for blame, and previous experiences of health care to reproductive autonomy in pregnancy decision making.

In these multiple ways, abortion became unchooseable for most of the women I interviewed, with the upshot that they had no real choice in their pregnancy decision making. Although I have not presented these findings as a comparison, there were geographical patterns in terms of what factors rendered abortion unchooseable. Specifically, more women in Louisiana described structural barriers, and specifically abortion restrictions, making abortion unchooseable. Given the higher number of state-level policies restricting abortion in Louisiana (Guttmacher Institute 2018a) compared to Maryland (Guttmacher Institute 2018b) at the time of data collection, this makes sense. Still, some Maryland women experienced structural barriers that made abortion unchooseable, and many Louisiana respondents described no structural contributors to abortion becoming unchooseable for them. Meanwhile, more Maryland women described how a previous medical experience of abortion contributed to anticipated negative embodiment of abortion, thereby making abortion unchooseable for this pregnancy. Given the characteristics of my sample, this, too, makes sense. More Maryland respondents than Louisiana respondents reported a prior abortion experience, which is a prerequisite for having an experience-based negative expectation for abortion. Still, some Louisiana respondents described anticipated negative embodiment of abortion, particularly regarding the conditions of care, rendering abortion unchooseable, and many of the Maryland respondents with a history of abortion did not find abortion unchooseable because of it.

Taken together, these findings demonstrate that constraints on pregnant women's reproductive autonomy are prevalent and not unique to states like Louisiana with numerous restrictive policies on abortion. While there is some geographic patterning in how abortion becomes unchooseable, that it becomes unchooseable is an experience women in both states shared, along with their low-income class status and, for most, a Black racial identity.

At a basic level, failure to recognize how abortion is unchooseable in respondents' pregnancy decision making is of concern because it disregards the lived experiences of these women. Given the chronic under-attention to women's lived experiences, and more specifically to the lived experiences of low-income and poor women and of women of color, attention to the specifics of their decision making alone has value. Further, this examination, by distinguishing and naming the structural, cultural, and experiential constraints that rendered abortion unchooseable, identifies where these constraints come from and who they affect. I show how autonomy in pregnancy decision making, for some, has become a raced and classed privilege. By uncovering the patterns across these women's experiences of how abortion came to be unchooseable, this book shows not only that reproductive autonomy is being constrained, but also how this is an effect of race, class, and gender inequality.

The women I interviewed were not without agency, even as, as I have demonstrated, their autonomy to make a pregnancy decision was compromised. Six respondents attempted to end their pregnancies on their own, either in response to structural barriers or anticipated negative embodiment of abortion rendering abortion unchooseable. They failed. In most cases, their efforts evidenced desperation. Still, they were actions taken, evidence of agency. Other respondents sought financial and/or emotional help from their social networks, trying to make abortion chooseable. They failed. Their efforts, too, were sometimes desperate. While they were not able to achieve their intended goals, these women did take action, resisting the constraints on their ability to make a pregnancy choice. Their agency, nonetheless, was limited. It was characterized by working with what they had rather than about being able to make a true pregnancy choice.

Their failures must be understood not as personal shortcomings but as evidence of the strength of the constraints on their autonomy. Without accurate information on how to end a pregnancy on their own or access to social networks with this information, respondents unsurprisingly did not deploy methods such as those Aiken and colleagues (2018) describe of procuring abortion pills to safely self-manage an abortion. Immersed in communities that were similarly financially struggling, respondents were predictably unsuccessful in securing financial resources. When their social networks also lacked alternative narratives of the meaning of abortion, they had no source of affirming narratives that could make abortion chooseable. Likewise, respondents were unlikely to learn from their networks about abortion funds, which help low-income pregnant people cover the costs of abortion as well as provide practical support such as transportation (National Network of Abortion Funds n.d.).

While my findings are specific to these respondents' accounts, there is reason to think that the abortion as unchooseable framework has utility beyond this sample. This analysis has revealed how race and class inequality contribute to abortion becoming unchooseable for socially marginalized populations, suggesting the transferability of these findings beyond these geographic settings to other low-income populations. Additionally, while this study centers how abortion becomes unchooseable for Black women, the white, biracial, and Hispanic respondents also gave accounts of abortion as unchooseable. When we focus on pregnancy decision making, rather than solely on pregnancy outcomes, we better understand the impediments to true reproductive autonomy—and where they come from.

The Origins and Perpetuation of Constrained Choice

Several of the processes making abortion unchooseable have occurred without broad public notice, and it is to these social processes that I turn now. Many of these processes owe to the antiabortion movement. Scholarship on the antiabortion movement has charted its tactics (Blanchard 1994; Haugeberg 2017; Hussey 2019), narrative frames (Ehrlich and Doan 2019; Mason 2002), and activists' histories (Ginsburg 1998; Luker 1984; Maxwell 2002; Munson 2008). Here, I have illustrated the on-the-ground impact of these efforts on women's lives. Certainly, policies championed by abortion opponents, consistent with extant literature (Cook et al. 1999; Jerman, Frohwirth, et al. 2017; S. Roberts, Johns, et al. 2019; Upadhyay, Weitz, et al. 2014), made abortion unchooseable for some respondents. Extending research on the impacts of the antiabortion movement, I further show how the antiabortion movement has developed and forwarded cultural narratives on the meaning of abortion that rendered abortion unchooseable for other respondents.

Scholars of social movements have considered how collective action frames can serve the political goals of a movement (Benford and Snow 2000). My analysis illustrates how collective action frames generated by the antiabortion movement that are used in public protests and legislative tactics, including that abortion is killing and that abortion harms women, constrain individual pregnancy decisions. Scholarship demonstrates that the pregnancy help movement (also known as the crisis pregnancy movement)—which Kelly (2014) identifies as the main source of the abortion as harmful narrative—has historically eschewed political action in favor of social change by targeting individual pregnant people (Hussey 2019). My data suggest that antiabortion cultural framings have succeeded in making abortion unchooseable for some women, even if there is no evidence that antiabortion pregnancy resource centers themselves change women's minds about abortion (Kimport, Kriz, and Roberts 2018). Potentially, this case offers insight into strategies of social movement–led culture change around abortion. Because respondents voiced few alternate narratives to the antiabortion cultural narratives on the meaning of abortion—and some voiced none, hearing only antiabortion cultural narratives from every source they sought—it is not clear whether these narratives made abortion unchooseable because they were more resonant than abortion-affirming narratives or because there simply were no alternative narratives in respondents' communities.

And yet, although the antiabortion movement succeeded in making abortion unchooseable through policy barriers and by dominating the discursive terms of the meaning of abortion, it was not the only source of abortion becoming unchooseable for respondents. For example, as I noted above, Louisiana's prohibition on public insurance coverage of abortion, which prevented some respondents from choosing abortion, was consequential because respondents—and their social networks—were financially struggling. The two-visit requirement became an obstacle for women who did not have flexibility in their work hours, which is a more common feature of low-wage work. Their low-income status, in other words, was what made these antiabortion policies consequential. This class status, as I have explained, is related to racist policies and practices that perpetuate wealth and income inequality by race (Baradaran 2017; Branch and Jackson 2020; Oliver and Shapiro 2006), contributing to patterns of limited class mobility (Laurison, Dow, and Chernoff 2020), rendering not only poverty but also structural racism a contributor to the potency of these antiabortion policies. Put differently, the antiabortion movement has succeeded in mobilizing policy restrictions to make abortion unchooseable for some pregnant people by leveraging existing class and race inequality. Following Holland's (2020) exposition of how the contemporary antiabortion movement in the United States is rooted in a white racial desire to reclaim moral authority lost with slavery and ongoing racism, racism may even be the unacknowledged source of persistent antiabortion identity.

The way that embodied experiences of health care influenced respondents' reproductive autonomy, too, is not exclusively an effect of the antiabortion movement's efforts. These women's distrust of medical professionals and negative past experiences of health care, including abortion, are part of a legacy of racist mistreatment of people of color by healthcare systems and individual providers (Dehlendorf et al. 2010; LaVeist, Rolley, and Diala 2003; Thorburn and Bogart 2005). These experiences exist outside of antiabortion efforts, even as they are available for being leveraged by antiabortion tactics.

What Would Reproductive Autonomy Look Like?

If I am arguing that abortion being unchooseable undermines some pregnant people's reproductive agency in pregnancy and parenting, one might ask: What would reproductive autonomy look like? And, more pointedly, what would reproductive autonomy look like for socially vulnerable populations? The factors my analysis has identified that make abortion unchooseable do not affect the population equally. Poverty and racism make low-income and poor women of color more vulnerable to the constraints on their pregnancy decision making I have delineated here. I start to answer this question of how to achieve reproductive autonomy for all by centering this population of women whose reproductive autonomy is currently negated.

True reproductive autonomy requires that abortion be something all pregnant people can choose. To be clear, this does not mean they will or have to choose abortion, only that abortion is a truly chooseable pregnancy outcome. From the experiences of the Louisiana respondents, it is clear that the absence of policies restricting public insurance coverage of abortion, the absence of a two-visit requirement, and the integration of abortion care into mainstream medicine would contribute to making abortion chooseable. The accounts of the Maryland respondents illustrate, further, that policies that reduce poverty could make abortion chooseable.

Looking at the experiences of respondents from both states together, cultural narratives that affirm abortion as a moral, responsible, and safe choice could make abortion chooseable. When respondents were unable to fathom how they could choose abortion, alternative narratives of the meaning of abortion might make choosing abortion possible. The elimination of racial discrimination and mistreatment by providers and the healthcare system could make abortion chooseable. When pregnant people trust that they will receive equitable care from healthcare providers, abortion can become chooseable.

Broadly, making abortion chooseable for every pregnant person requires attending to and dismantling the structural and cultural barriers I have documented. It requires centering the desires and circumstances of individual pregnant people, and addressing their concerns, fears, and needs. Perhaps most importantly, to the extent that processes rendering abortion unchooseable rest on other forms of systemic oppression, including race, class, and gender, reproductive autonomy for all cannot be accomplished so long as those systems of oppression remain.

Reproductive autonomy, however, is about more than making abortion chooseable. Although I have argued that when abortion is unchooseable, reproductive agency and autonomy are negated, making abortion chooseable is necessary but not sufficient to ensure real pregnancy choice. True reproductive autonomy also means that having a baby is a chooseable pregnancy outcome. As described in chapter 5, some respondents reported being pressured into a previous abortion, illustrating an instance we could understand as having-a-baby-as-unchooseable. True reproductive autonomy means ensuring that all pregnancy outcomes are chooseable for all pregnant people, regardless of their income, race, or other characteristics. It means affirming low-income and poor women's and women of color's right to parent.

Finally, it must be stated that reproductive autonomy alone is not enough to achieve true reproductive justice. Following reproductive justice principles (Ross and Solinger 2017), people have the right to determine whether and when to parent as well as to raise their children in safe and sustainable communities. Although this analysis has focused on reproductive autonomy in pregnancy decision making, or lack thereof, readers will have noticed how prevalent violence was in the lives of the women I interviewed. This violence took multiple forms. Many described experiences of unsafe neighborhoods and homelessness that are part of the broader structural violence of underinvestment in low-income communities and communities of color. Even more described personal experiences of physical and emotional abuse, both in their past and ongoing. None of the factors that made abortion unchooseable contributed to ensuring that these women could parent in safe and sustainable communities. And true reproductive justice demands safe and sustainable communities.

The accounts of the women I interviewed of why they considered and did not obtain an abortion reveal deep constraints on their reproductive autonomy, even for those who continued their pregnancies because they wanted to have a baby. Their experiences detail a chronic and consequential injustice that is specific to their social location as low-income and poor Black women. We would not know any of this without their honest, immensely thoughtful, and sometimes heartbreaking accounts. I thank them for sharing their stories. We owe them real choice.

Methodological Appendix

Between June 2015 and June 2017, my colleague Sarah Roberts and I conducted a mixed methods study that recruited pregnant people presenting for their first prenatal appointment (see also S. Roberts, Kimport, et al. 2019 for a summary of methods). Sarah spearheaded the quantitative portions of the study, including site selection, in-clinic data collection, and quantitative analysis; I led the qualitative portions, including sampling strategy, phone interview data collection, and qualitative analysis. Sarah deserves the credit for the clever overarching study design. The study was designed to examine people's needs, resources, and decision making in pregnancy, with attention to barriers to abortion care. The study protocols were approved by the University of California, San Francisco Institutional Review Board and the Louisiana State University Health Sciences Campus Institutional Review Board. The University of Maryland Institutional Review Board relied on the approval of the University of California, San Francisco Institutional Review Board.

Site Selection

The study started recruitment in Louisiana, a state with numerous laws on the books regulating abortion. Louisiana is regularly considered by advocates both supportive of and opposed to abortion rights to be hostile to abortion. We recruited from three prenatal clinics in southern Louisiana. To offer a quantitative comparison to the experiences in Louisiana, a short while into that recruitment, we began recruitment in a second state: Maryland. We selected Maryland because it is a state with few regulations of abortion and high service availability, thereby enabling a comparison to Louisiana, for which neither was true. Within Maryland, we chose to recruit in Baltimore because the city had the same racial and financial demographics as the areas we were recruiting from in southern Louisiana, and the specific site we recruited from in Baltimore, too, served patients with racial and financial demographics similar to those served by the sites in Louisiana.

Recruitment

At each study site, an on-site research coordinator approached all patients over age eighteen who spoke English and were presenting for their first prenatal care appointment. Although we did not screen for gender identity, we assume based on interpersonal conversations on-site that all who participated identified as cisgender women. Accordingly, inferences made about pregnant people in this book are intentionally limited to cisgender women. About six months into the first year of recruitment, we expanded eligibility criteria to include Spanish-speaking patients. Clinic staff alerted the research coordinator to eligible potential participants, who then screened them for eligibility. Clinic patients who were under eighteen, were not pregnant, had already received prenatal care at the facility, did not speak or read English or Spanish, or were incarcerated were not eligible. (Pregnant people who are incarcerated often receive their care outside of the jail or prison where they are held. For more about this, see the excellent work of physician and anthropologist Carolyn Sufrin [2017].) Interested and eligible potential participants completed written informed consent.

At their clinic visit, participants completed a quantitative data collection that had two parts. First, they completed a self-administered iPad survey. The survey included questions about their demographics, the circumstances of their current pregnancy (including partner, pregnancy intention, initial and current pregnancy outcome preference), pregnancy history, general health, and alcohol and drug use. After participants completed the self-administered survey, they then completed a structured in-clinic interview with the research coordinator. Depending on their survey responses, the in-clinic interview lasted between five and fifteen minutes. The structured interview included desired health and social services, experiences with antiabortion pregnancy resource centers (also known as crisis pregnancy centers), actions taken toward obtaining an abortion, reasons for not obtaining an abortion, and, in the Maryland data collection only, interest in and use of alcohol and drug use disorder treatment during this pregnancy. In both quantitative data collection modes, we asked participants the following question: "Did you consider having an abortion during this pregnancy even for one second?" Upon completing these activities, participants received a $30 gift card to a major retail vendor.

The research coordinators approached 747 potential participants. A total of 559 completed both modes of data collection, 269 in Louisiana and 290 in Maryland. The sample size was determined by calculations based on quantitative analyses of interest. Recruitment ceased when that size was reached.

For the qualitative component of the data collection, a subset of participants was invited to complete an in-depth interview by phone between one and three weeks after the in-clinic collection. I conducted all phone interviews. Among the motivating research questions for the qualitative data collection was the question of why people consider but do not obtain an abortion. We were initially unsure whether people would accurately report their answers to the question in the quantitative data collection about whether they considered abortion, so we created expansive in-depth interview inclusion criteria: have completed the in-clinic data collections and reported considering abortion, presented for prenatal care after the first trimester, or reported that the pregnancy was unintended. (For a separate research question, we recruited participants who reported visiting a pregnancy resource center. There was little overlap between visiting a center and considering abortion.) The latter two criteria were established with the expectation that delay in presentation for prenatal care may have been due to consideration of abortion and the assumption that abortion is more commonly considered for unintended pregnancies than intended pregnancies. After I completed seven interviews with Louisiana respondents who were eligible because of these latter two criteria, we dropped them as eligibility criteria. None of those seven women had considered abortion, suggesting that those inclusion criteria were not useful. Maryland recruitment took place after this narrowed eligibility frame, but we applied the more expansive inclusion criteria to include seven women who did not report considering abortion to confirm that the criteria were likewise not useful in that setting.

As data collection progressed, the inclusion criteria were further narrowed to ensure that more rare experiences were captured in the sample. In specific, after recruiting about twenty-five respondents in each state, we narrowed the inclusion criteria to not only reporting having considered abortion but also having taken at least one action toward obtaining an abortion (including any report of attempting to end the pregnancy on their own). The final month of data collection was curtailed as the emotional toll of data collection was too high and burnout imminent (see Dickson-Swift et al. 2007 for discussion of challenges to researchers in conducting research on sensitive topics). One interview was canceled (and remuneration for the respondent's time still given), and follow-up procedures for missed interviews became laxer. Interview respondents were offered a $50 gift card to a major retailer as remuneration for their time. Respondents had the option to have the gift card mailed to them or to pick it up directly from the on-site research coordinator at their recruitment site.

Interview Format

Interviews were conducted by phone. This decision was made intentionally for several reasons. Scholars have argued that phone modality for interviews can afford greater feeling of anonymity for participants, especially related to sensitive topics (Greenfield, Midanik, and Rogers 2000). We anticipated that feelings of anonymity might make the respondent feel more comfortable sharing potentially very private experiences. Conducting the interviews by phone also enabled the project to capture interview data from both Louisiana and Maryland respondents concurrently. It was also lower cost than conducting in-person interviews at multiple sites would be, especially over the two-year recruitment period the project needed.

During data collection, I identified several additional advantages for this project of the phone modality. I found that phone interviews enabled respondents to complete the interview in a larger range of locations than an in-person interview would allow. Most respondents spoke with me from their homes, but some talked to me from parks, their cars, a relative's or friend's home, the waiting room of a hospital, or a Walmart as she did her shopping—and some moved between several locations during the interview. Similarly, while most respondents were alone when I interviewed them, a substantial number were supervising their children, and some had other adults nearby for all or part of the interview. I believe that meeting respondents where they were increased their trust in me and, for several, enabled them to participate when they would not have been able to otherwise (e.g., because there was no alternative caregiver for their children or because they lacked reliable transportation).

Conducting the interviews by phone did pose some difficulties. I had difficulty understanding several respondents and they me, sometimes because of difference in accent, sometimes because of the quality of our connection, and sometimes because of the respondent's mumbling, using speakerphone, or not speaking directly into the phone. I think these challenges would have been less pronounced in person. Additionally, many interviews were interrupted, both by tasks the respondent was undertaking (e.g., driving) and by other people nearby (e.g., children requesting a snack). In a handful of instances, respondents asked me to call them back another time, which I did. Broadly, I did not feel that these interruptions diminished rapport. Respondents conveyed commitment to the interview and focus on the interview questions, for example telling children who interrupted that they were on an important call. Finally, the phone format also meant I could not assess body language or capture respondents' presentation of self. I could, however, attend to their verbal inflections and pauses, and by not having a visual knowledge of them, my interviewing was arguably less susceptible to my own implicit biases. As their presentation of self was not a focal part of the research question, I do not think my inability to observe it was a significant concern for the validity of this analysis.

Throughout the data collection, respondents articulated that they enjoyed participating in the interviews, that they appreciated getting to talk about their experience, and that they were grateful to talk to someone who did not judge them. Several told me they liked getting to talk to a stranger about their experience. I found the interviews very rewarding to conduct. I also found the data collection emotionally difficult at times. I became upset during some interviews when the respondent was herself upset and describing her experience. In some interviews, I paused the interview to state to the respondent that her emotions were welcome and that I did not judge them and that she did not have to discuss anything that she did not want to. (I should note that other interviews were very upbeat, with several interviewees who made me laugh.) I think the phone format allowed my emotional response to some respondents' accounts to be less visible and, in that way, reduced the intrusion of my emotions on their stories. Such an intrusion both would represent an inappropriate burden on respondents and could have implications for the data itself, affecting what the respondent decided to share. Cumulatively, the emotional intensity of the interviews over two years led me to feel that burnout was imminent and data collection needed to stop. I discovered public health scientist Virginia Dickson-Swift and colleagues' (2007) article on the challenges for qualitative researchers conducting research on sensitive topics, and it rang true.

Interviews were semi-structured, allowing respondents to introduce topics as they felt appropriate. In addition to demographic characteristics, interviews included questions about the respondent's experience of entering prenatal care, the circumstances of her pregnancy, her reproductive history, and her knowledge of and position on abortion. In conducting the interviews, I followed the cues of the respondent, for example in her language about the man involved in her pregnancy, and strove to be non-judgmental and non-corrective. I did not correct scientifically inaccurate statements, though I did not necessarily convey agreement. I aimed to be empathetic and affirming of respondents' ability to make the right decision for their pregnancy for themselves. On more than one occasion, after a respondent had shared an experience of mistreatment by someone else (including sexual partners, parents or guardians, family members, and healthcare workers), I told them I was sorry that had happened and that I thought they deserved to be treated with love and respect. These are basic behaviors of having a conversation with another person but are not always considered appropriate in "research." I did them anyway.

When asked, I shared honest information about myself and my beliefs. As stated in chapter 1, my social location differed in several ways from that of most respondents, most notably in my race (white), age (older than nearly every respondent at the time of data collection), and employment (employed full time in a white-collar profession, i.e., as an academic), which could be understood as a proxy of my class status. The only characteristic respondents asked me about was whether I was a parent. I responded truthfully that I am. It bears noting that the phone format may have enabled some of these differences to be less obvious (e.g., age) or affected respondents' ability to ask me about myself. Some respondents mistakenly thought I was employed by the prenatal care site where they were recruited. When references to me being part of the hospital or clinic came up in interviews, I corrected this misunderstanding and clarified that anything they shared with me would not be directly shared back to the hospital/clinic or have any effect on the care they received at the hospital/clinic.

I completed interviews with forty-three women in Louisiana, twenty-eight of whom reported considering abortion for this pregnancy, between June 2015 and May 2017. I completed interviews with forty women in Maryland, thirty of whom reported considering abortion for this pregnancy, between November 2016 and June 2017. Interviews ranged in length from about thirty minutes to an hour and forty-five minutes, averaging just under one hour. There was no difference in average interview length by recruitment state. Interviews were audio recorded and transcribed by a professional transcription service.

Respondent Characteristics

In the full quantitative sample, we found that about 30 percent of participants had considered abortion for this pregnancy (S. Roberts, Kimport, et al. 2019). That makes consideration of abortion rather common. When we drilled into predictors of consideration of abortion, we found that participants reporting greater economic insecurity and more mental health diagnoses or substance use had higher odds of having considered abortion (S. Roberts, Berglas, and Kimport 2020). Certainly, it may be that the rate of considering abortion is lower in other populations, such as among people who intended to become pregnant or those with greater economic security. Nonetheless, this finding shows that consideration of abortion is relatively common—and, importantly, the rate of consideration of abortion was not statistically different among pregnant people in two states with different regulations and availability of abortion care.

Before delving into the characteristics of the interview respondents, I note that, while the quantitative components of the study were designed to enable comparison, it was not a rationale in the interview data collection. We recruited respondents purposively, endeavoring to capture a range of experiences. The interviews aimed to illuminate patterns that may be influenced by geography but are not exclusive to one geographical area or another.

The interview respondents analyzed in the book (that is, the fifty-eight women who reported considering abortion for this pregnancy) ranged in age from eighteen to thirty-eight, with an average age of twenty-seven. Most respondents identified as Black and/or African American (86%; N = 50), with three who identified as Hispanic in Louisiana, two in each state who identified as white, and one woman in Maryland who identified as Black and Mexican. Most identified as religious (64%; N = 37), naming Christianity or a form of Christianity (e.g., Baptist) as their religion. They were all struggling financially. More than half were unemployed (55%; N = 32), and most relied on a form of public health insurance (83%; N = 48) or were uninsured (14%; N = 8). In terms of highest educational attainment, 17 percent (N = 10) had not completed high school; 41 percent (N = 24) had completed high school or its equivalent; 38 percent (N = 22) had completed some college; and just one woman in each state had completed a four-year college degree or more (3%; N = 2).

Respondents from the two states differed systematically from one another only regarding their pregnancy history. More Louisiana respondents had never given birth than Maryland respondents: 39 percent (N = 11) of Louisiana respondents were nulliparous compared to just 17 percent (N = 5) of Maryland respondents. Additionally, Maryland respondents had more children in their household: 63 percent (N = 19) of Maryland respondents had two or more children compared to 39 percent (N = 11) of Louisiana respondents. Finally, more than twice as many Maryland respondents had a history of abortion (67%; N = 20) compared to Louisiana respondents (25%; N = 7).

Analysis

I took extensive field notes after every interview, and these notes served as my first analysis of the data. When all interviews were complete, I wrote detailed summaries of each interviewee's experience, noting when and whether they considered abortion, adoption, and parenting for this pregnancy as well as the personal, interpersonal, institutional, and policy-related challenges to abortion and to having a baby they were navigating. From these summaries, I wrote memos on patterns within each state's interviews and across the full sample.

I wrote several memos on the patterns related to race and class in the interviews. When we began recruitment in Louisiana, the study goal of the interviews was to understand pregnancy decision making in a state with numerous policies related to abortion—not pregnancy decision making of a specific racial group. That is, I did not set out to focus on Black women. Nor did I intend to focus specifically on low-income and poor women. As recruitment began, though, I quickly discovered that it was low-income and poor women and Black women who, in that geographical area, were presenting to prenatal care having considered but not obtained an abortion. The attention to race and class in the analysis, then, was emergent rather than part of the interview study design.

Drawing on my field notes and the summaries, I developed a preliminary codebook. I applied the codebook to three transcripts from each state, adding emergent codes. When I felt that the codebook was sufficient, I coded all fifty-eight transcripts using Atlas.ti 7. Consistent with abductive analysis (Timmermans and Tavory 2012), this analysis was iterative and both deductive and inductive, deepened through ongoing immersion in the literature, conversations with other scholars, and collaborations with the study team.

Deidentification

All names in this book are pseudonyms. In assigning pseudonyms, I aimed to protect respondents' real identities while retaining some of the age, geography, and race signifiers of given names. With the invaluable research assistance of Erin Wingo, I developed a list of pseudonyms that were common to women of Black, Hispanic, and white ancestry born in the 1980s, 1990s, and 2000s using records from websites including those of the Social Security

Administration and BabyCenter. We ensured that the names were not similar to or nicknames of the real names of any of the eighty-three interviewees in the larger study. Pseudonyms were then assigned to all respondents, with effort to have pseudonyms align with respondents' birth decade, geography, and self-identified race.

To ensure deidentification, there are instances in this book where I have generalized aspects of respondents' medical conditions or pregnancy history. For example, I note that some respondents had medical conditions, but when the specific condition was unique enough to be identifying, I do not specify the condition. When a condition is common—either in the general population or among pregnant people—I have retained specificity. However, even with a common condition or pregnancy experience, if other aspects of the respondent's experience when combined with knowledge of that condition could be identifying, I generalized the condition or the pregnancy history.

Acknowledgments

Above all else, I thank the women whose accounts are the foundation of this analysis for their time and trust. I learned from them in ways I could not have anticipated. In this book, I strive to fulfill the responsibility to honor the accounts of their lived experience they entrusted me with.

As nearly every book acknowledgments section notes, scholarship is always a collaborative endeavor. The scholarship in this book would not have been possible without Sarah C. M. Roberts, who generously allowed me to piggyback a qualitative component on the ambitious quantitative Multistate Abortion Prenatal Study she led. I thank Sarah for her brilliant study design and implementation and invaluable insights into this analysis. I thank everyone who worked on the Multistate Abortion Prenatal Study, Finley Baba, Elise Belusa, Nancy Berglas, Anna Bernstein, Mattie Boehler-Tatman, Ivette Gomez, Heather Gould, Jenny Holl, Rebecca Kriz, Heather Lipkovich, Katrina Mark, Nicole Nguyen, Brenly Rowland, Alison Swiatlo, Ushma Upadhyay, Valerie Williams, and Erin Wingo, for their vital help with data collection as well as for research and project assistance. I thank the facilities in Louisiana and Maryland for their collaboration. This book also would not have been possible without the support of the David and Lucile Packard Foundation and an anonymous foundation. The sponsors had no involvement in study design; in the collection, analysis, and interpretation of data; or in the decision to write this book.

In the course of writing this book, I benefited from the time, insight, encouragement, and knowledge of colleagues near and far.

For this, I thank Krystale Littlejohn always. I thank Erin Wingo, Danielle Bessett, Katherine Ehrenreich, Isabel Muñoz, Jeanne Flavin, Tracy Weitz, Antonia Biggs, Corrine Rocca, and Lori Freedman for brainstorming with me and offering excellent feedback. On specific subject areas, it was an immense privilege to be able to go directly to people with deep knowledge, and I am grateful to them for their generosity. For this, I thank Jill Adams, Angel Foster, Heather Gould, Daniel Grossman, Rachel K. Jones, Lauren McIvor Thompson, and Ushma Upadhyay. What I get wrong in this book is despite their efforts.

I am forever grateful to my colleagues past and present in the Advancing New Standards in Reproductive Health (ANSIRH) program of the Bixby Center for Global Reproductive Health and the University of California, San Francisco. You are my academic home, and I am indebted to you for your humor, engagement, intelligence, and commitment to justice. Thank you for teaching me and for learning with me.

I thank Peter Mickulas, my Rutgers University Press editor, for his enthusiasm for this project from the beginning and the academic editors of the Families in Focus series, particularly Nazli Kibria, for their thoughtful review of the manuscript. No author could ask for better support.

Finally, I thank my family David, Barbara, Rebecca, and Sam Kimport for their unconditional love and support and Matthew Villeneuve and our children, Mathilde and Viola, for the love and joy they bring to my life.

References

Adler, Nancy E., and Katherine Newman. 2002. "Socioeconomic Disparities in Health: Pathways and Policies." *Health Affairs* 21 (2): 60–76.

Aiken, Abigail R. A., Kathleen Broussard, Dana M. Johnson, and Elisa Padron. 2018. "Motivations and Experiences of People Seeking Medication Abortion Online in the United States." *Perspectives on Sexual and Reproductive Health* 50 (4): 157–163.

Alexander, Michelle. 2020. *The New Jim Crow: Mass Incarceration in the Age of Colorblindness*. New York: The New Press.

Allen, Mallary. 2014. "Narrative Diversity and Sympathetic Abortion: What Online Storytelling Reveals about the Prescribed Norms of the Mainstream Movements." *Symbolic Interaction* 38 (1): 42–63.

American College of Obstetricians and Gynecologists. 2013. "ACOG Practice Bulletin No. 135: Second-Trimester Abortion." *Obstetrics & Gynecology* 121 (6): 1394–1406.

Ammerman, Nancy Tatom. 1990. *Baptist Battles: Social Change and Religious Conflict in the Southern Baptist Convention*. New Brunswick, NJ: Rutgers University Press.

Anachebe, Ngozi F., and Madeline Y. Sutton. 2003. "Racial Disparities in Reproductive Health Outcomes." *American Journal of Obstetrics and Gynecology* 188 (4): S37–S42.

Andaya, Elise, and Joanna Mishtal. 2017. "The Erosion of Rights to Abortion Care in the United States: A Call for a Renewed Anthropological Engagement with the Politics of Abortion." *Medical Anthropology Quarterly* 31 (1): 40–59.

APA Task Force on Mental Health and Abortion. 2008. *Report of the APA Task Force on Mental Health and Abortion*. Washington, DC: American Psychological Association.

Artiga, Samantha, Kendal Orgera, and Anthony Damico. 2020. "Changes in Health Coverage by Race and Ethnicity since the ACA, 2010–2018." Retrieved March 15, 2020. https://www.kff.org/disparities-policy/issue-brief/changes-in-health-coverage-by-race-and-ethnicity-since-the-aca-2010-2018/.

Balasubramanian, Bijal A., Kitaw Demissie, Benjamin F. Crabtree, Pamela A. Ohman Strickland, Karen Pawlish, and George G. Rhoads. 2012. "Black Medicaid Beneficiaries Experience Breast Cancer Treatment Delays More Frequently Than Whites." *Ethnicity and Disease* 22 (3): 288–294.

Baradaran, Mehrsa. 2017. *The Color of Money: Black Banks and the Racial Wealth Gap*. Cambridge, MA: Harvard University Press.

Becker, Davida, and Amy O. Tsui. 2008. "Reproductive Health Service Preferences and Perceptions of Quality among Low-Income Women: Racial, Ethnic and Language Group Differences." *Perspectives on Sexual and Reproductive Health* 40 (4): 202–211.

Bélanger, Eliane, Ronald Melzack, and Pierre Lauzon. 1989. "Pain of First-Trimester Abortion: A Study of Psychosocial and Medical Predictors." *Pain* 36 (3): 339–350.

Benford, Robert, and David A. Snow. 2000. "Framing Processes and Social Movements: An Overview and Assessment." *Annual Review of Sociology* 26:611–639.

Bensonsmith, Dionne. 2005. "Jezebels, Matriarchs, and Welfare Queens: The Moynihan Report of 1965 and the Social Construction of African-American Women in Welfare Policy." In *Deserving and Entitled: Social Constructions and Public Policy*, edited by Anne L. Schneider and Helen M. Ingram, 243–259. Albany: State University of New York Press.

Berglas, Nancy F., Molly F. Battistelli, Wanda K. Nicholson, Mindy Sobota, Richard D. Urman, and Sarah C. M. Roberts. 2018. "The Effect of Facility Characteristics on Patient Safety, Patient Experience, and Service Availability for Procedures in Non-Hospital-Affiliated Outpatient Settings: A Systematic Review." *PLOS One* 13 (1): e0190975.

Berglas, Nancy F., Heather Gould, David K. Turok, Jessica N. Sanders, Alissa C. Perrucci, and Sarah C. M. Roberts. 2017. "State-Mandated (Mis)Information and Women's Endorsement of Common Abortion Myths." *Women's Health Issues* 27 (2): 129–135.

Bertotti, Andrea M. 2013. "Gendered Divisions of Fertility Work: Socioeconomic Predictors of Female versus Male Sterilization." *Journal of Marriage and Family* 75:13–25.

Biggs, M. Antonia, Heather Gould, and Diana Greene Foster. 2013. "Understanding Why Women Seek Abortions in the US." *BMC Women's Health* 13 (1): 29.

Biggs, M. Antonia, Ushma D. Upadhyay, Charles E. McCulloch, and Diana G. Foster. 2017. "Women's Mental Health and Well-Being 5 Years after Receiving or Being Denied an Abortion: A Prospective, Longitudinal Cohort Study." *JAMA Psychiatry* 74 (2): 169–178.

Blanchard, Dallas A. 1994. *The Anti-Abortion Movement and the Rise of the Religious Right: From Polite to Fiery Protest.* New York: Twayne.

Boonstra, Heather, Vanessa Duran, Vanessa Northington Gamble, Paul Blumenthal, Linda Dominguez, and Cheri Pies. 2000. "The 'Boom and Bust Phenomenon': The Hopes, Dreams, and Broken Promises of the Contraceptive Revolution." *Contraception* 61 (1): 9–25.

Borrero, Sonya, Nikki Zite, Joseph E. Potter, and James Trussell. 2014. "Medicaid Policy on Sterilization—Anachronistic or Still Relevant?" *New England Journal of Medicine* 370 (2): 102.

Boyd, Rhea W., Edwin G. Lindo, Lachelle D. Weeks, and Monica R. McLemore. 2020. "On Racism: A New Standard for Publishing on Racial Health Inequities." *Health Affairs Blog* 10. doi: 10.1377/hblog20200630.939347.

Branch, Enobong Hannah, and Christina Jackson. 2020. *Black in America: The Paradox of the Color Line.* Medford, MA: Polity Press.

Bridges, Khiara. 2011. *Reproducing Race: An Ethnography of Pregnancy as a Site of Racialization.* Berkeley: University of California Press.

Casper, Monica. 1998. *The Making of the Unborn Patient: A Social Anatomy of Fetal Surgery.* New Brunswick, NJ: Rutgers University Press.

Clark, Rodney, Norman B. Anderson, Vernessa R. Clark, and David R. Williams. 1999. "Racism as a Stressor for African Americans: A Biopsychosocial Model." *American Psychologist* 54 (10): 805.

Cockrill, Kate, and Adina Nack. 2013. "'I'm Not That Type of Person': Managing the Stigma of Having an Abortion." *Deviant Behavior* 34:973–990.

Cohen, David S., and Carole Joffe. 2020. *Obstacle Course: The Everyday Struggle to Get an Abortion in America*. Berkeley: University of California Press.

Collins, Patricia Hill. 2006. *From Black Power to Hip Hop: Racism, Nationalism, and Feminism*. Philadelphia: Temple University Press.

Conradt, Elisabeth, Tess Flannery, Judy L. Aschner, Robert D. Annett, Lisa A. Croen, Cristiane S. Duarte, Alexander M. Friedman, Constance Guille, Monique M. Hedderson, and Julie A. Hofheimer. 2019. "Prenatal Opioid Exposure: Neurodevelopmental Consequences and Future Research Priorities." *Pediatrics* 144 (3): e20190128.

Cook, Philip J., Allan M. Parnell, Michael J. Moore, and Deanna Pagnini. 1999. "The Effects of Short-Term Variation in Abortion Funding on Pregnancy Outcomes." *Journal of Health Economics* 18 (2): 241–257.

Daniels, Cynthia R. 2008. *Exposing Men: The Science and Politics of Male Reproduction*. New York: Oxford University Press.

D'Anna, Laura Hoyt, Marissa Hansen, Brittney Mull, Carol Canjura, Esther Lee, and Stephanie Sumstine. 2018. "Social Discrimination and Health Care: A Multidimensional Framework of Experiences among a Low-Income Multiethnic Sample." *Social Work in Public Health* 33 (3): 187–201.

Dehlendorf, Christine, Maria Isabel Rodriguez, Kira Levy, Sonya Borrero, and Jody Steinauer. 2010. "Disparities in Family Planning." *American Journal of Obstetrics and Gynecology* 202 (3): 214–220.

Desai, Sheila, Rachel K. Jones, and Kate Castle. 2018. "Estimating Abortion Provision and Abortion Referrals among United States Obstetrician-Gynecologists in Private Practice." *Contraception* 97 (4): 297–302.

Desmond, Matthew. 2016. *Evicted: Poverty and Profit in the American City*. New York: Broadway Books.

Dickson-Swift, Virginia, Erica L. James, Sandra Kippen, and Pranee Liamputtong. 2007. "Doing Sensitive Research: What Challenges Do Qualitative Researchers Face?" *Qualitative Research* 7 (3): 327–353.

Doan, Alesha E. 2007. *Opposition and Intimidation: The Abortion Wars and Strategies of Political Harassment*. Ann Arbor: University of Michigan Press.

Doan, Alesha E., and Corinne Schwarz. 2020. "Father Knows Best: 'Protecting' Women through State Surveillance and Social Control in Anti-abortion Policy." *Politics and Policy* 48 (1): 6–37.

Downing, Roberta A., Thomas A. LaVeist, and Heather E. Bullock. 2007. "Intersections of Ethnicity and Social Class in Provider Advice regarding Reproductive Health." *American Journal of Public Health* 97 (10): 1803–1807.

Drew, Elaine M., and Nancy E. Schoenberg. 2011. "Deconstructing Fatalism: Ethnographic Perspectives on Women's Decision Making about Cancer Prevention and Treatment." *Medical Anthropology Quarterly* 25 (2): 164–182.

Dubow, Sara. 2010. *Ourselves Unborn: A History of the Fetus in Modern America*. New York: Oxford University Press.

Duster, Troy. 2003. *Backdoor to Eugenics*. New York: Routledge.

Ebrahim, Shahul H., John E. Anderson, Rosaly Correa-de-Araujo, Samuel F. Posner, and Hani K. Atrash. 2009. "Overcoming Social and Health Inequalities among U.S. Women of Reproductive Age—Challenges to the Nation's Health in the 21st Century." *Health Policy* 90 (2–3):196–205.

Edin, Kathryn, and Maria Kefalas. 2011. *Promises I Can Keep: Why Poor Women Put Motherhood before Marriage*. Berkeley: University of California Press.

Ehrlich, J. Shoshanna, and Alesha E. Doan. 2019. *Abortion Regret: The New Attack on Reproductive Freedom*. Santa Barbara: ABC-CLIO.

Esnaola, Nestor F., and Marvella E. Ford. 2012. "Racial Differences and Disparities in Cancer Care and Outcomes: Where's the Rub?" *Surgical Oncology Clinics* 21 (3): 417–437.

Fennell, Julie Lynn. 2011. "Men Bring Condoms, Women Take Pills: Men's and Women's Roles in Contraceptive Decision Making." *Gender and Society* 25 (4): 496–521.

Finer, Lawrence B., Lori F. Frohwirth, Lindsay A. Dauphinee, Susheela Singh, and Ann M. Moore. 2005. "Reasons U.S. Women Have Abortions: Quantitative and Qualitative Perspectives." *Perspectives on Sexual and Reproductive Health* 37 (3): 110–118.

Finer, Lawrence B., and Mia R. Zolna. 2016. "Declines in Unintended Pregnancy in the United States, 2008–2011." *New England Journal of Medicine* 374 (9): 843–852.

Flavin, Jeanne. 2008. *Our Bodies, Our Crimes: The Policing of Women's Reproduction in America*. New York: New York University Press.

Flavin, Jeanne, and Lynn M. Paltrow. 2010. "Punishing Pregnant Drug-Using Women: Defying Law, Medicine, and Common Sense." *Journal of Addictive Diseases* 29 (2): 231–244.

Foster, Diana Greene, Heather Gould, J. Taylor, and T. A. Weitz. 2012. "Attitudes and Decision-Making among Women Seeking Abortion at One U.S. Clinic." *Perspectives on Sexual and Reproductive Health* 44 (2): 117–124.

Foster, Diana Greene, Katrina Kimport, Heather Gould, Sarah C. Roberts, and Tracy A. Weitz. 2013. "Effect of Abortion Protesters on Women's Emotional Response to Abortion." *Contraception* 87 (1): 81–87. doi: 10 .1016/j.contraception.2012.09.005.

Frank, Peter, Roseanne Mcnamee, Philip C. Hannaford, Clifford R. Kay, and Sybil Hirsch. 1993. "The Effect of Induced Abortion on Subsequent Fertility." *BJOG: An International Journal of Obstetrics and Gynaecology* 100 (6): 575–580.

Freedman, Lori R. 2010. *Willing and Unable: Doctors' Constraints in Abortion Care*. Nashville: Vanderbilt University Press.

Fuentes, Liza, and Jenna Jerman. 2019. "Distance Traveled to Obtain Clinical Abortion Care in the United States and Reasons for Clinic Choice." *Journal of Women's Health* 28 (12): 1623–1631.

Gamble, Vanessa Northington. 1997. "Under the Shadow of Tuskegee: African Americans and Health Care." *American Journal of Public Health* 87 (11): 1773–1778.

Gee, Gilbert C., and Devon C. Payne-Sturges. 2004. "Environmental Health Disparities: A Framework Integrating Psychosocial and Environmental Concepts." *Environmental Health Perspectives* 112 (17): 1645–1653.

Gelman, Amanda, Elian A. Rosenfeld, Cara Nikolajski, Lori R. Freedman, Julia R. Steinberg, and Sonya Borrero. 2017. "Abortion Stigma among Low-Income Women Obtaining Abortions in Western Pennsylvania: A Qualitative Assessment." *Perspectives on Sexual and Reproductive Health* 49 (1): 29–36.

Ginsburg, Faye D. 1998. *Contested Lives: The Abortion Debate in an American Community*. Berkeley: University of California Press.

Ginsburg, Faye D., and Rayna Rapp. 1995. *Conceiving the New World Order: The Global Politics of Reproduction*. Berkeley: University of California Press.

Gordon, Linda. 2002. *The Moral Property of Women: A History of Birth Control Politics in America*. Chicago: University of Illinois Press.

Greenfield, Thomas K., Lorraine T. Midanik, and John D. Rogers. 2000. "Effects of Telephone versus Face-to-Face Interview Modes on Reports of Alcohol Consumption." *Addiction* 95 (2): 277–284.

Greil, Arthur L., Julia McQuillan, Karina M. Shreffler, Katherine M. Johnson, and Kathleen S. Slauson-Blevins. 2011. "Race-Ethnicity and Medical Services for Infertility: Stratified Reproduction in a Population-Based Sample of U.S. Women." *Journal of Health and Social Behavior* 52 (4): 493–509.

Grossman, Daniel, Kate Grindlay, Anna L. Altshuler, and Jay Schulkin. 2019. "Induced Abortion Provision among a National Sample of Obstetrician-Gynecologists." *Obstetrics and Gynecology* 133 (3): 477–83.

Grossman, Daniel, Kari White, Kristine Hopkins, and Joseph E. Potter. 2017. "Change in Distance to Nearest Facility and Abortion in Texas, 2012 to 2014." *JAMA* 317 (4): 437–439.

Guttmacher Institute. 2018a. "State Facts about Abortion: Louisiana." Retrieved July 31, 2018. https://www.guttmacher.org/fact-sheet/state -facts-about-abortion-louisiana.

———. 2018b. "State Facts about Abortion: Maryland." Retrieved July 31, 2018. https://www.guttmacher.org/fact-sheet/state-facts-about -abortion-maryland.

Halva-Neubauer, Glen A., and Sara L. Zeigler. 2010. "Promoting Fetal Personhood: The Rhetorical and Legislative Strategies of the Pro-Life Movement after *Planned Parenthood v. Casey*." *Feminist Formations* 22 (2): 101–123.

Haraway, Donna. 1988. "Situated Knowledges: The Science Question in Feminism and the Privilege of Partial Perspective." *Feminist Studies* 14 (3): 575–599.

Haugeberg, Karissa. 2017. *Women against Abortion: Inside the Largest Moral Reform Movement of the Twentieth Century*. Urbana: University of Illinois Press.

Heslin, Kevin C., Ronald M. Andersen, Susan L. Ettner, and William E. Cunningham. 2005. "Racial and Ethnic Disparities in Access to Physicians with HIV-Related Expertise: Findings from a Nationally Representative Study." *Journal of General Internal Medicine* 20 (3): 283–289.

Higgins, Jenny A., and Nicole K. Smith. 2016. "The Sexual Acceptability of Contraception: Reviewing the Literature and Building a New Concept." *Journal of Sex Research* 53 (4–5): 417–456.

Hoffman, Kelly M., Sophie Trawalter, Jordan R. Axt, and M. Norman Oliver. 2016. "Racial Bias in Pain Assessment and Treatment Recommendations, and False Beliefs about Biological Differences between Blacks and Whites." *Proceedings of the National Academy of Sciences* 113 (16): 4296–4301.

Hoffmann, John P., and Sherrie Mills Johnson. 2005. "Attitudes toward Abortion among Religious Traditions in the United States: Change or Continuity?" *Sociology of Religion* 66 (2): 161–182.

Holland, Jennifer L. 2020. *Tiny You: A Western History of the Anti-Abortion Movement*. Berkeley: University of California Press.

House Committee on Oversight and Reform. n.d. "Planned Parenthood Fact v. Fiction." Retrieved September 17, 2020. https://oversight.house.gov/planned-parenthood-fact-v-fiction.

Hull, N.E.H., and Peter Charles Hoffer. 2010. *Roe v. Wade: The Abortion Rights Controversy in American History*. Lawrence: University Press of Kansas.

Hussey, Laura S. 2019. *The Pro-Life Pregnancy Help Movement: Serving Women or Saving Babies?* Lawrence: University Press of Kansas.

Jackson, Andrea V., Deborah Karasek, Christine Dehlendorf, and Diana Greene Foster. 2016. "Racial and Ethnic Differences in Women's Preferences for Features of Contraceptive Methods." *Contraception* 93 (5): 406–411.

Jerman, Jenna, Lori Frohwirth, Megan L. Kavanaugh. and Nakeisha Blades. 2017. "Barriers to Abortion Care and Their Consequences for Patients Traveling for Services: Qualitative Findings from Two States." *Perspectives on Sexual and Reproductive Health* 49 (2): 95–102.

Jerman, Jenna, Rachel K. Jones, and Tsuyoshi Onda. 2016. "Characteristics of U.S. Abortion Patients in 2014 and Changes since 2008." New York:

Guttmacher Institute. Retrieved March 23, 2020. https://www
.guttmacher.org/report/characteristics-us-abortion-patients-2014.

Joffe, Carole. 1995. *Doctors of Conscience: The Struggle to Provide Abortion before and after Roe v. Wade*. Boston: Beacon Press.

Jones, Rachel K., Meghan Ingerick, and Jenna Jerman. 2018. "Differences in Abortion Service Delivery in Hostile, Middle-Ground, and Supportive States in 2014." *Women's Health Issues* 28 (3): 212–218.

Jones, Rachel K., and Jenna Jerman. 2017. "Population Group Abortion Rates and Lifetime Incidence of Abortion: United States, 2008–2014." *American Journal of Public Health* 107 (12): 1904–1909.

Jones, Rachel K., Elizabeth Witwer, and Jenna Jerman. 2019. "Abortion Incidence and Service Availability in the United States, 2017." New York: Guttmacher Institute. Retrieved April 22, 2020. https://www
.guttmacher.org/report/abortion-incidence-service-availability-us-2017.

Jozkowski, Kristen N., Brandon L. Crawford, and Mary E. Hunt. 2018. "Complexity in Attitudes toward Abortion Access: Results from Two Studies." *Sexuality Research and Social Policy* 15 (4): 464–482.

Kelly, Kimberly. 2012. "In the Name of the Mother: Renegotiating Conservative Women's Authority in the Crisis Pregnancy Center Movement." *Signs* 38 (1): 203–230.

———. 2014. "The Spread of 'Post Abortion Syndrome' as Social Diagnosis." *Social Science and Medicine* 102:18–25.

Kessler, Ronald C., Kristin D. Mickelson, and David R. Williams. 1999. "The Prevalence, Distribution, and Mental Health Correlates of Perceived Discrimination in the United States." *Journal of Health and Social Behavior* 40 (3): 208–230.

Kieltyka, Lyn, Pooja Mehta, Karis Schoellmann, and Chloe Lake. 2018, "Louisiana Maternal Mortality Review Report, 2011–2016." Retrieved October 27, 2020. https://ldh.la.gov/assets/oph/Center-PHCH/Center
-PH/maternal/2011-2016_MMR_Report_FINAL.pdf.

Killen, Kimberly. 2019. "'Can You Hear Me Now?' Race, Motherhood, and the Politics of Being Heard." *Politics and Gender* 15 (4): 623–644.

Kimport, Katrina. 2012. "(Mis)Understanding Abortion Regret." *Symbolic Interaction* 35 (2): 105–122.

———. 2018a. "More Than a Physical Burden: Women's Mental and Emotional Work in Preventing Pregnancy." *Journal of Sex Research* 55 (9): 1096–1105.

———. 2018b. "Talking about Male Body-Based Contraceptives: The Counseling Visit and the Feminization of Contraception." *Social Science and Medicine* 201:44–50.

———. 2019. "Pregnant Women's Experiences of Crisis Pregnancy Centers: When Abortion Stigmatization Succeeds and Fails." *Symbolic Interaction* 42 (4): 618–639.

———. 2020. "Pregnant Women's Reasons for and Experiences of Visiting Antiabortion Pregnancy Resource Centers." *Perspectives on Sexual and Reproductive Health* 52 (1): 49–56.

Kimport, Katrina, and Colin Doty. 2019. "Interpreting the Truth: How People Make Sense of New Information about Abortion." *Women's Health Issues* 29 (2): 182–187.

Kimport, Katrina, Kira Foster, and Tracy Weitz. 2011. "Social Sources of Women's Emotional Difficulty after Abortion: Lessons from a Qualitative Analysis of Women's Abortion Narratives." *Perspectives on Sexual and Reproductive Health* 43 (2): 103–109.

Kimport, Katrina, and Lori R. Freedman. 2018. "Abortion: A Most Common Deviance." In *Routledge Handbook of Deviance*, edited by Stephen E. Brown and Ophir Sefiha, 221–231. New York: Routledge.

Kimport, Katrina, Nicole E. Johns, and Ushma D. Upadhyay. 2018. "Coercing Women's Behavior: How a Mandatory Viewing Law Changes Patients' Preabortion Ultrasound Viewing Practices." *Journal of Health Politics, Policy and Law* 43 (6): 941–960.

Kimport, Katrina, Rebecca Kriz, and Sarah C. M. Roberts. 2018. "The Prevalence and Impacts of Crisis Pregnancy Center Visits among a Population of Pregnant Women." *Contraception* 98 (1): 69–73.

Kimport, Katrina, and Brenly Rowland. 2017. "Taking Insurance in Abortion Care: Policy, Practices, and the Role of Poverty." *Research in the Sociology of Health Care* 35:39–57.

Kumar, Anuradha, Leila Hessini, and Ellen M. H. Mitchell. 2009. "Conceptualising Abortion Stigma." *Culture, Health and Sexuality* 11 (6): 1–15.

Laurison, Daniel, Dawn Dow, and Carolyn Chernoff. 2020. "Class Mobility and Reproduction for Black and White Adults in the United States: A Visualization." *Socius* 6:1–3. doi:10.1177/2378023120960959.

LaVeist, Thomas A., Lydia A. Isaac, and Karen Patricia Williams. 2009. "Mistrust of Health Care Organizations Is Associated with Underutilization of Health Services." *Health Services Research* 44 (6): 2093–2105.

LaVeist, Thomas A., Nicole C. Rolley, and Chamberlain Diala. 2003. "Prevalence and Patterns of Discrimination among U.S. Health Care Consumers." *International Journal of Health Services* 33 (2): 331–344.

Lavin, Maud. 2001. *Clean New World: Culture, Politics, and Graphic Design*. Cambridge, MA: MIT Press.

Layne, Linda. 2000. "'He Was a Real Baby with Baby Things': A Material Culture Analysis of Personhood, Parenthood and Pregnancy Loss." *Journal of Material Culture* 5 (3): 321–345.

———. 2003. *Motherhood Lost: A Feminist Account of Pregnancy Loss in America*. New York: Routledge.

Lessard, Lauren N., Deborah Karasek, Sandi Ma, Philip Darney, Julianna Deardorff, Maureen Lahiff, Dan Grossman, and Diana Greene Foster. 2012. "Contraceptive Features Preferred by Women at High Risk of Unintended Pregnancy." *Perspectives on Sexual and Reproductive Health* 44 (3): 194–200.

Link, Bruce G., and Jo C. Phelan. 2001. "Conceptualizing Stigma." *Annual Review of Sociology* 27 (1): 363–385.

Littlejohn, Krystale E. 2012. "Hormonal Contraceptive Use and Discontinuation Because of Dissatisfaction: Differences by Race and Education." *Demography* 49 (4): 1433–1452.

———. 2021. *Just Get on the Pill: The Uneven Burden of Reproductive Politics*. Berkeley: University of California Press.

Littlejohn, Krystale E., and Katrina Kimport. 2017. "Contesting and Differentially Constructing Uncertainty: Negotiations of Contraceptive Use in the Clinical Encounter." *Journal of Health and Social Behavior* 58 (4): 442–454.

Ludlow, Jeannie. 2008. "Sometimes, It's a Child *and* a Choice: Toward an Embodied Abortion Praxis." *NWSA Journal* 20 (1): 26–50.

Luker, Kristin. 1975. *Taking Chances: Abortion and the Decision Not to Contracept*. Berkeley: University of California Press.

———. 1984. *Abortion and the Politics of Motherhood*. Berkeley: University of California Press.

Luna, Zakiya, and Kristin Luker. 2013. "Reproductive Justice." *Annual Review of Law and Social Science* 9:327–352.

Mann, Emily S. 2013. "Regulating Latina Youth Sexualities through Community Health Centers: Discourses and Practices of Sexual Citizenship." *Gender and Society* 27 (5): 681–703.

Mann, Emily S., Ashley L. White, Peyton L. Rogers, and Anu Manchikanti Gomez. 2019. "Patients' Experiences with South Carolina's Immediate Postpartum Long-Acting Reversible Contraception Medicaid Policy." *Contraception* 100 (2): 165–171.

Maryland Department of Health and Mental Hygiene. 2017. "Maryland Maternal Mortality Review: 2016 Annual Report." Retrieved October 2, 2020. https://phpa.health.maryland.gov/Documents /Maryland-Maternal-Mortality-Review-2016-Report.pdf.

Mason, Carol. 2002. *Killing for Life: The Apocalyptic Narrative of Pro-Life Politics*. Ithaca, NY: Cornell University Press.

Maxwell, Carol J. C. 2002. *Pro-Life Activists in America*. New York: Cambridge University Press.

McCaffrey, Dawn, and Jennifer Keys. 2000. "Competitive Framing Processes in the Abortion Debate: Polarization-Vilification, Frame Saving, and Frame Debunking." *Sociological Quarterly* 41 (1): 41–61.

McGowan, Michelle L., Alison H. Norris, and Danielle Bessett. 2020. "Care Churn—Why Keeping Clinic Doors Open Isn't Enough to Ensure Access to Abortion." *New England Journal of Medicine* 383 (6): 508–510.

Meyer, David, and Suzanne Staggenborg. 2008. "Opposing Movement Strategies in U.S. Abortion Politics." *Research in Social Movements, Conflicts and Change* 28:207–238.

Mitchell, Lisa M., and Eugenia Georges. 1998. "Baby's First Picture." In *Cyborg Babies: From Techno-sex to Techno-tots*, edited by Robbie Davis-Floyd and Joseph Dumit, 105–124. New York: Routledge.

Mohr, James C. 1979. *Abortion in America: The Origins and Evolution of National Policy*. Oxford: Oxford University Press.

Morgan, Lynn. 2009. *Icons of Life: A Cultural History of Human Embryos*. Berkeley: University of California Press.

Morgan, Lynn Marie, and Meredith W. Michaels. 1999. *Fetal Subjects, Feminist Positions*. Philadelphia: University of Pennsylvania Press.

Morgan, M. 2004. "The Payment of Drug Addicts to Increase Their Sterilisation Rate Is Morally Unjustified and Not Simply 'a Fine Balance.'" *Journal of Obstetrics and Gynaecology* 24 (2): 119–123.

Moseson, Heidi, Stephanie Herold, Sofia Filippa, Jill Barr-Walker, Sarah E. Baum, and Caitlin Gerdts. 2020. "Self-Managed Abortion: A Systematic Scoping Review." *Best Practice and Research: Clinical Obstetrics and Gynaecology* 63:87–110.

Munson, Ziad W. 2008. *The Making of Pro-Life Activists: How Social Movement Mobilization Works*. Chicago: University of Chicago Press.

Nadasen, Premilla. 2007. "From Widow to 'Welfare Queen': Welfare and the Politics of Race." *Black Women, Gender and Families* 1 (2): 52–77.

Nash, Elizabeth. 2020. "State Abortion Policy Landscape: From Hostile to Supportive." Retrieved October 27, 2020. https://www.guttmacher.org /article/2019/08/state-abortion-policy-landscape-hostile-supportive.

Nash, Elizabeth, and Rachel Benson Gold. 2015. "In Just the Last Four Years, States Have Enacted 231 Abortion Restrictions." Retrieved October 27, 2020. https://www.guttmacher.org/article/2015/01/just -last-four-years-states-have-enacted-231-abortion-restrictions#.

National Academies of Sciences, Engineering and Medicine. 2018. *The Safety and Quality of Abortion Care in the United States*. Washington, DC: National Academies Press.

National Network of Abortion Funds. n.d. "National Network of Abortion Funds." Retrieved October 27, 2020. https://abortionfunds .org/about/.

Nelson, Jennifer. 2003. *Women of Color and the Reproductive Rights Movement*. New York: New York University Press.

Nickerson, Adrianne, Ruth Manski, and Amanda Dennis. 2014. "A Qualitative Investigation of Low-Income Abortion Clients' Attitudes toward Public Funding for Abortion." *Women and Health* 54 (7): 672–686.

Norris, Alison, Danielle Bessett, Julia R. Steinberg, Megan L. Kavana-ugh, Silvia De Zordo, and Davida Becker. 2011. "Abortion Stigma: A Reconceptualization of Constituents, Causes, and Consequences." *Women's Health Issues* 21 (3S): S49–S54.

Oaks, Laury. 2001. *Smoking and Pregnancy: The Politics of Fetal Protection*. New Brunswick, NJ: Rutgers University Press.

O'Connor, Annette M., Peter Tugwell, George A Wells, Tom Elmslie, Elaine Jolly, Garry Hollingworth, Ruth McPherson, Helen Bunn, Ian Graham, and Elizabeth Drake. 1998. "A Decision Aid for Women Considering Hormone Therapy after Menopause: Decision Support Framework and Evaluation." *Patient Education and Counseling* 33 (3): 267–279.

O'Donnell, Jenny, Alisa Goldberg, Ellice Lieberman, and Theresa Betancourt. 2018. "'I Wouldn't Even Know Where to Start': Unwanted Pregnancy and Abortion Decision-Making in Central Appalachia." *Reproductive Health Matters* 26 (54): 98–113.

O'Donnell, Jenny, Tracy A. Weitz, and Lori R. Freedman. 2011. "Resistance and Vulnerability to Stigmatization in Abortion Work." *Social Science and Medicine* 73 (9): 1357–1364. doi: 10.1016/j.socscimed.2011.08.019.

Ojanuga, Durrenda. 1993. "The Medical Ethics of the 'Father of Gynaecology', Dr J Marion Sims." *Journal of Medical Ethics* 19 (1): 28–31.

Oliver, Melvin L., and Thomas M. Shapiro. 2006. *Black Wealth, White Wealth: A New Perspective on Racial Inequality*. New York: Routledge.

Owens, Deirdre Cooper. 2017. *Medical Bondage: Race, Gender, and the Origins of American Gynecology*. Athens: University of Georgia Press.

Penney, Gillian. 2006. "Treatment of Pain during Medical Abortion." *Contraception* 74 (1): 45–47.

Petchesky, Rosalind P. 1984. *Abortion and Woman's Choice: The State, Sexuality, and Reproductive Freedom*. New York: Longman.

———. 1987. "Fetal Images: The Power of Visual Culture in the Politics of Reproduction." *Feminist Studies* 13 (2): 263–292.

Polletta, Francesca, Pang Ching Bobby Chen, Beth Gharrity Gardner, and Alice Motes. 2011. "The Sociology of Storytelling." *Annual Review of Sociology* 37:109–130.

Purcell, Carrie. 2015. "The Sociology of Women's Abortion Experiences: Recent Research and Future Directions." *Sociology Compass* 9 (7): 585–596.

Raymond, Elizabeth G., Daniel Grossman, Mark A. Weaver, Stephanie Toti, and Beverly Winikoff. 2014. "Mortality of Induced Abortion,

Other Outpatient Surgical Procedures and Common Activities in the United States." *Contraception* 90 (5): 476–479.

Reagan, Leslie J. 1997. *When Abortion Was a Crime: Women, Medicine, and Law in the United States, 1867–1973.* Berkeley: University of California Press.

Renner, Regina-Maria, Jeffrey T. J. Jensen, Mark D. N. Nichols, and Alison Edelman. 2009. "Pain Control in First Trimester Surgical Abortion." *Cochrane Database of Systematic Reviews*, no. 2, CD006712. doi: 10.1002/14651858.CD006712.pub2.

Roberts, Dorothy E. 1999. *Killing the Black Body: Race, Reproduction, and the Meaning of Liberty.* New York: Vintage.

Roberts, Sarah C. M., Nancy F. Berglas, and Katrina Kimport. 2020. "Complex Situations: Economic Insecurity, Mental Health, and Substance Use among Pregnant Women Who Consider—but Do Not Have—Abortions." *PLOS One* 15 (1): e0226004.

Roberts, Sarah C. M., Heather Gould, Katrina Kimport, Tracy A. Weitz, and Diana Greene Foster. 2014. "Out-of-Pocket Costs and Insurance Coverage for Abortion in the United States." *Women's Health Issues* 24 (2): e211–e218.

Roberts, Sarah C. M., Nicole E. Johns, Valerie Williams, Erin Wingo, and Ushma D. Upadhyay. 2019. "Estimating the Proportion of Medicaid-Eligible Pregnant Women in Louisiana Who Do Not Get Abortions When Medicaid Does Not Cover Abortion." *BMC Women's Health* 19 (1): 78.

Roberts, Sarah C. M., Katrina Kimport, Rebecca Kriz, Jennifer Holl, Katrina Mark, and Valerie Williams. 2019. "Consideration of and Reasons for Not Obtaining Abortion among Women Entering Prenatal Care in Southern Louisiana and Baltimore, Maryland." *Sexuality Research and Social Policy* 1 6(4): 476–487.

Roberts, Sarah C. M., David K. Turok, Elise Belusa, Sarah Combellick, and Ushma D. Upadhyay. 2016. "Utah's 72-Hour Waiting Period for Abortion: Experiences among a Clinic-Based Sample of Women." *Perspectives on Sexual and Reproductive Health* 48 (4): 179–187.

Roberts, Sarah C. M., Ushma D. Upadhyay, Guodong Liu, Jennifer L. Kerns, Djibril Ba, Nancy Beam, and Douglas L. Leslie. 2018. "Association of Facility Type with Procedural-Related Morbidities and Adverse

Events among Patients Undergoing Induced Abortions." *JAMA* 319 (24): 2497–2506.

Roberts, Sarah C. M., Erin Wingo, and Katrina Kimport. 2020. "A Qualitative Exploration of Women's Experiences Discovering Pregnancies in the Emergency Department." *Contraception: X*, 2 (2002): 100024. doi: 10.1016/j.conx.2020.100024.

Rocca, Corinne H., Katrina Kimport, Heather Gould, and Diana Greene Foster. 2013. "Women's Emotions One Week after Receiving or Being Denied an Abortion." *Perspectives on Sexual and Reproductive Health* 45 (3): 122–131.

Rocca, Corinne H., Katrina Kimport, Sarah C. M. Roberts, Heather Gould, John Neuhaus, and Diana G. Foster. 2015. "Decision Rightness and Emotional Responses to Abortion in the United States: A Longitudinal Study." *PLOS One* 10 (7). doi: 10.1371/journal. pone.0128832.

Rocca, Corinne H., Goleen Samari, Diana G. Foster, Heather Gould, and Katrina Kimport. 2020. "Emotions and Decision Rightness over Five Years following an Abortion: An Examination of Decision Difficulty and Abortion Stigma." *Social Science and Medicine* 248 (March). doi: 10.1016/j.socscimed.2019.112704.

Rohlinger, Deana A. 2002. "Framing the Abortion Debate: Organizational Resources, Media Strategies, and Movement-Countermovement Dynamics." *Sociological Quarterly* 43 (4): 479–507.

———. 2006. "Friends and Foes: Media, Politics, and Tactics in the Abortion War." *Social Problems* 53 (4): 537–561.

———. 2015. *Abortion Politics, Mass Media, and Social Movements in America*. New York: Cambridge University Press.

Rosenthal, Lisa, and Marci Lobel. 2016. "Stereotypes of Black American Women Related to Sexuality and Motherhood." *Psychology of Women Quarterly* 40 (3): 414–427.

Ross, Loretta, Erika Derkas, Whitney Peoples, Lynn Roberts, and Pamela Bridgewater. 2017. *Radical Reproductive Justice: Foundation, Theory, Practice, Critique*. New York: Feminist Press at CUNY.

Ross, Loretta, and Rickie Solinger. 2017. *Reproductive Justice: An Introduction*. Vol. 1. Berkeley: University of California Press.

Roth, Rachel, and Sara L. Ainsworth. 2015. "'If They Hand You a Paper, You Sign It': A Call to End the Sterilization of Women in Prison." *Hastings Women's Law Journal* 26:7.

Sanger, Carol. 2016. "Talking about Abortion." *Social and Legal Studies* 25 (6): 651–666.

Schoen, Johanna. 2005. *Choice and Coercion: Birth Control, Sterilization, and Abortion in Public Health and Welfare*. Chapel Hill: University of North Carolina Press.

———. 2015. *Abortion after Roe*. Chapel Hill: University of North Carolina Press.

Siegel, Reva B. 2008. "The Right's Reasons: Constitutional Conflict and the Spread of Woman-Protective Antiabortion Argument." *Duke Law Journal* 57:1641–1692.

Silbergeld, Ellen K., and Thelma E Patrick. 2005. "Environmental Exposures, Toxicologic Mechanisms, and Adverse Pregnancy Outcomes." *American Journal of Obstetrics and Gynecology* 192 (5): S11–S21.

Sisson, Gretchen, and Katrina Kimport. 2016. "Facts and Fictions: Characters Seeking Abortion on American Television, 2005–2014." *Contraception* 93 (5): 446–451.

Smith, Tom W., and Jaesok Son. 2013. "Trends in Public Attitudes towards Abortion." *General Social Survey 2012 Final Report*. Retrieved April 7, 2020. https://www.norc.org/PDFs/GSS%20Reports/Trends%20 in%20Attitudes%20About%20Abortion_Final.pdf.

Smith-Rosenberg, Carroll. 1986. *Disorderly Conduct: Visions of Gender in Victorian America*. Oxford University Press on Demand.

Solazzo, Alexa L. 2019. "Different and Not Equal: The Uneven Association of Race, Poverty, and Abortion Laws on Abortion Timing." *Social Problems* 66 (4): 519–547.

Steinberg, Julia R., Davida Becker, and Jillian T. Henderson. 2011. "Does the Outcome of a First Pregnancy Predict Depression, Suicidal Ideation, or Lower Self-Esteem? Data from the National Comorbidity Survey." *American Journal of Orthopsychiatry* 81 (2): 193–201.

Stern, Alexandra Minna. 2005. "Sterilized in the Name of Public Health: Race, Immigration, and Reproductive Control in Modern California." *American Journal of Public Health* 95 (7): 1128–1138.

Stevens, Lindsay M. 2015. "Planning Parenthood: Health Care Providers' Perspectives on Pregnancy Intention, Readiness, and Family Planning." *Social Science and Medicine* 139 (2015): 44–52.

Stormer, Nathan. 2015. *Sign of Pathology: U.S. Medical Rhetoric on Abortion, 1800s–1960s.* University Park: Pennsylvania State University Press.

Sufrin, Carolyn. 2017. *Jailcare: Finding the Safety Net for Women behind Bars.* Berkeley: University of California Press.

Swidler, Ann. 2001. *Talk of Love: How Culture Matters.* Chicago: University of Chicago Press.

Taylor, Janelle S. 1992. "The Public Fetus and the Family Car: From Abortion Politics to a Volvo Advertisement." *Public Culture* 4 (2): 67–80.

———. 2008. *The Public Life of the Fetal Sonogram: Technology, Consumption, and the Politics of Reproduction.* New Brunswick, NJ: Rutgers University Press.

Thomas, Susan L. 1998. "Race, Gender, and Welfare Reform: The Antinatalist Response." *Journal of Black Studies* 28 (4): 419–446.

Thorburn, Sheryl, and Laura M. Bogart. 2005. "African American Women and Family Planning Services: Perceptions of Discrimination." *Women and Health* 42 (1): 23–39.

Timmermans, Stefan, and Iddo Tavory. 2012. "Theory Construction in Qualitative Research: From Grounded Theory to Abductive Analysis." *Sociological Theory* 30 (3): 167–186.

Torres, Aida, and Jacqueline Darroch Forrest. 1988. "Why Do Women Have Abortions?" *Family Planning Perspectives* 20 (4): 169–176.

Upadhyay, Ushma D., Sheila Desai, Vera Zlidar, Tracy A. Weitz, Daniel Grossman, Patricia Anderson, and Diana Taylor. 2015. "Incidence of Emergency Department Visits and Complications after Abortion." *Obstetrics and Gynecology* 125 (1): 175–183.

Upadhyay, Ushma D., Katrina Kimport, Elise Belusa, Nicole E. Johns, Douglas W. Laube, and Sarah C. M. Roberts. 2017. "Evaluating the Impact of a Mandatory Pre-abortion Ultrasound Viewing Law: A Mixed Methods Study." *PLOS One* 12 (7): e0178871. doi: 10.1371/journal.pone.0178871.

Upadhyay, Ushma D., Tracy A. Weitz, Rachel K. Jones, Rana E. Barar, and Diana Greene Foster. 2014. "Denial of Abortion because of Provider

Gestational Age Limits in the United States." *American Journal of Public Health* 104(9):1687–1694.

Vaisey, Stephen. 2009. "Motivation and Justification: A Dual-Process Model of Culture in Action." *American Journal of Sociology* 114 (6): 1675–1715.

Van der Sijpt, Erica. 2014. "Complexities and Contingencies Conceptualised: Towards a Model of Reproductive Navigation." *Sociology of Health and Illness* 36 (2): 278–290.

Washington, Harriet A. 2006. *Medical Apartheid: The Dark History of Medical Experimentation on Black Americans from Colonial Times to the Present*. New York: Doubleday Books.

Weitz, Tracy A., and Katrina Kimport. 2012. "A Need to Expand Our Thinking about 'Repeat' Abortions." *Contraception* 85 (4): 408–412. doi: 10.1016/j.contraception.2011.09.003.

———. 2015. "The Discursive Production of Abortion Stigma in the Texas Ultrasound Viewing Law." *Berkeley Journal of Gender, Law and Justice* 30 (1): 6–21.

White, Kari, Sarah E. Baum, Kristine Hopkins, Joseph E. Potter, and Daniel Grossman. 2019. "Change in Second-Trimester Abortion after Implementation of a Restrictive State Law." *Obstetrics and Gynecology* 133 (4): 771.

Wilcox, Allen J., David B. Dunson, Clarice R. Weinberg, James Trussell, and Donna Day Baird. 2001. "Likelihood of Conception with a Single Act of Intercourse: Providing Benchmark Rates for Assessment of Post-Coital Contraceptives." *Contraception* 63 (4): 211–215.

Wilcox, Brian L., Jennifer K. Robbennolt, Janet E. O'Keeffe, and Marisa E Pynchon. 1996. "Teen Nonmarital Childbearing and Welfare: The Gap between Research and Political Discourse." *Journal of Social Issues* 52 (3): 71–90.

Williams, Clare, Priscilla Alderson, and Bobbie Farsides. 2001. "Conflicting Perceptions of the Fetus: Person, Patient, 'Nobody,' Commodity?" *New Genetics and Society* 20 (3): 225–238.

Williams, Daniel K. 2015a. *Defenders of the Unborn: The Pro-Life Movement before Roe v. Wade*. Oxford: Oxford University Press.

———. 2015b. "The Partisan Trajectory of the American Pro-Life Movement: How a Liberal Catholic Campaign Became a Conservative Evangelical Cause." *Religions* 6 (2): 451–475.

Woodruff, Katie. 2019. "Coverage of Abortion in Select U.S. Newspapers." *Women's Health Issues* 29 (1): 80–86.

World Health Organization Department of Reproductive Health and Research (WHO/RHR) and Johns Hopkins Bloomberg School of Public Health/Center for Communication Programs (CCP), INFO Project. 2007. *Family Planning: A Global Handbook for Providers.* Baltimore: CCP and WHO.

Ziegler, Mary. 2015. *After Roe: The Lost History of the Abortion Debate.* Cambridge, MA: Harvard University Press.

Index

About the Author

KATRINA KIMPORT is an associate professor in the Department of Obstetrics, Gynecology, and Reproductive Sciences and a research sociologist with the Advancing New Standards in Reproductive Health (ANSIRH) program of the Bixby Center for Global Reproductive Health at the University of California, San Francisco. Her research examines the (re)production of social inequality, with a particular focus on gender, health, and reproduction. She is the author of *Queering Marriage: Challenging Family Formation in the United States* and co-author of *Digitally Enabled Social Change*.

Printed in the United States
by Baker & Taylor Publisher Services